Chronic Fatigue Syndrome/ME

SUPPORT FOR FAMILY AND FRIENDS
Series Editors: Joanne Kerr and Alison Welsby

When a family member or friend is chronically ill or has a life-altering condition, not knowing how best to help can make you feel helpless. However, there are simple things that you can do to help both the person affected and the main carer (if this isn't you). The Support for Family and Friends series has been created for this purpose: to help you help your loved ones.

Providing up-to-date information about the illness or condition, as well as enabling you to understand what your family member or friend is going through, each book offers a wide range of ideas and advice about how to help, what to say and what to do. A useful directory of support groups and sources of information is also included so that you can access the best resources out there. You will be left feeling well informed and empowered to help – even if just to offer peace and quiet – in the most welcome and appropriate way.

of related interest

Managing Depression with Qigong
Frances Gaik
ISBN 978 1 84819 018 4

Chronic Fatigue Syndrome/ME

SUPPORT FOR FAMILY AND FRIENDS

ELIZABETH TURP

Jessica Kingsley *Publishers*
London and Philadelphia

First published in 2011
by Jessica Kingsley Publishers
116 Pentonville Road
London N1 9JB, UK
and
400 Market Street, Suite 400
Philadelphia, PA 19106, USA

www.jkp.com

Library of Congress Cataloging in Publication Data
Turp, Elizabeth.
Chronic fatigue syndrome/ME : support for family and friends / Elizabeth Turp.
p. cm. -- (Support for family and friends)
Includes bibliographical references and index.
ISBN 978-1-84905-141-5 (alk. paper)
1. Chronic fatigue syndrome--Popular works. I. Title.
RB150.F37T87 2010
616'.0478--dc22
2010012801

British Library Cataloguing in Publication Data
A CIP catalogue record for this book is available from the British Library

ISBN 978 1 84905 141 5

Printed and bound in the United States by
Thomson-Shore, Inc.

Contents

ACKNOWLEDGEMENTS   7

Introduction   9
  Why I have written this book and who it is for   9
  My story   11
  The different levels of CFS/ME: mild, moderate and severe   12
  The whole person: CFS/ME, the body and the mind   14

Chapter 1 What is Chronic Fatigue
Syndrome/ME?   17
  The different names for CFS/ME   17
  The symptoms   20
  The different stages of CFS/ME   23
  What does it feel like to have CFS/ME?   28
  Why has my friend/relative with CFS/ME not discussed
    this with me?   33
  How is it diagnosed?   36
  What causes CFS/ME?   41
  Treatment and management strategies   46
  Conclusion   50

Chapter 2 CFS/ME and You (the Friend or
Family Member)   51
  Your reaction to the news   52
  Changes in your relationship with the sufferer   64
  Being the main carer   68
  Partner relationships   69
  Brothers and sisters   74
  Parents   75
  Children   76

Friends 77
Colleagues 79
Communication 83
Support for you (the friend or family member) 93
Conclusion 96

Chapter 3 Supporting your Loved One to Cope with CFS/ME 97

Helping with the physical symptoms 98
Helping with the cognitive symptoms 108
Helping with the emotional effects 112
Other factors that make coping with CFS/ME harder 122
Helping with making positive changes: treatments and
    management strategies 125
Preventing relapse and staying stable 145
Other things that can help 149
Conclusion 152

Chapter 4 Practical Advice on How You Can Help with Everyday Life 153

Personal hygiene 154
Food and nutrition 156
Shopping 163
Mobility and travel 168
Domestic tasks, DIY and gardening 176
Money, employment and work 179
Caring responsibilities 185
Socialising and communication 187
Conclusion 197

Chapter 5 The Top Ten Tips on How You Can Help 199

Final note from the author 206

REFERENCES 207

RESOURCES 209

INDEX 236

Acknowledgements

I would like to thank everyone who has contributed their experiences and ideas to this book, and Action for ME, the Wellies Network and Stockport ME Group for helping to collect these. Thank you to John and Caroline and series editors Alison and Joanne for making this happen. My gratitude goes to Milon, Sairah, Betty, Mary, May, Paul and Anne-Marie for your skilled input. Many thanks to Don, Jo, Doreen and my family for your continuous enthusiasm and support throughout the process of writing.

Special thanks go to Jenny, Sandra, Fran, Pauline, Dr Nye, Dr Hulse and Paula for giving me what I needed to get to this point.

This book is dedicated to my partner Ed who has done all the above and so much more.

Introduction

WHY I HAVE WRITTEN THIS BOOK AND WHO IT IS FOR

This book has been written to help people who have a friend or family member with chronic fatigue syndrome/myalgic encephalomyelitis (CFS/ME) understand and support them, as well as help the sufferer themselves comprehend and cope with the effect the illness has had on them. People with CFS/ME experience extreme fatigue and many other symptoms including pain, headaches, impaired concentration, memory problems, anxiety, malaise, sleep problems and palpitations. CFS/ME is a complex, variable and serious disabling condition that affects all areas of a sufferer's life and, in turn, those close to them. Yet it is often misunderstood. In some areas there is little support available for sufferers, and even less for their friends and families. Health professionals such as home helps, care staff, counsellors, therapists, doctors and nurses supporting people who have CFS/ME may also find the contents of this book useful to widen their understanding of the complexity of the condition and deal with some of the difficulties that can arise in what to do and say. This book aims to increase awareness and understanding about the condition and by doing so help people with the illness too. Sufferers will, it is hoped, find this book a useful way of introducing subjects that are difficult to talk about or explain. It covers the practical, emotional, social and medical aspects of the illness and it is hoped that friends and family members and other care givers will find useful suggestions and advice on how they can help in a way that suits them.

This book is about adults with CFS/ME and while it is acknowledged that some of the information is relevant to children and young people, their needs are very different and merit a separate book written specifically for them.

The quotations and case studies included in this book come from personal contributions of people who have CFS/ME as well as friends and family of sufferers. People with the illness were asked 'What would you like people to do, say, know or understand about your life with CFS/ME?' Friends and family members were asked what they wished they had known and what they consider to be important issues for someone in their position. This invaluable research was done with the kind assistance of the British CFS/ME charity Action for ME, the Wellies Network (www.wellies. me.uk), a website run by recovering sufferers, and Stockport ME Group, a Cheshire-based UK support organisation. Details of these organisations and others can be found in the Resources section. It is acknowledged that people who have severe CFS/ME have found it more difficult to contribute but several people who have been severely affected in the past, and are now improved or recovered, have been able to put their experiences forward. I should also add that there are more female voices than male in the book because twice as many women as men are diagnosed with the illness. Some contributors have chosen to remain anonymous so that they could speak freely about their difficulties, and are referred to by pseudonyms indicated by quotation marks.

I would like to take this opportunity to thank everyone who has spent their time and often limited energy sending me powerful, emotive and resonant pieces about their experiences, making this book a rich source of information and support for others.

MY STORY

When I was seriously ill with CFS/ME, I found it incredibly difficult to find accurate or positive information to help me or the people around me, understand and cope with the illness. I have been to hell and back again. I was so ill I thought I would lose my friends, my home, the job I love as well as my sanity. At my worst I could hardly walk or stand up without holding on to something. I couldn't work, suffered severely disturbed sleep, couldn't open jars of food, couldn't concentrate on reading, had aching legs that made me cry, had to give up driving, sat on buses feeling so sick I nearly had to get off, and regularly broke down emotionally from the fear and frustration of what was happening to me. At times I was very difficult to be around and it was hard for people to support me for a lot of reasons. While I have been writing, friends and family members have told me that their own confusion and lack of knowledge about the illness was a big barrier for them. This is why I wanted to write this book: to pass on what I have learned from having CFS/ME. Whether you are a friend, a family member, carer, professional or someone with CFS/ME, I hope this book provides some of the support and advice I wish my loved ones and I had had easy access to.

Nowadays I am living a slower and less pressured life than before I was ill, having recovered most of my health. One of the lessons that CFS/ME has taught me is that life is short and looking after myself is now more of a priority. CFS/ME is a horrendous illness that can rob sufferers of relationships, financial security, self-esteem, the opportunity to feel a sense of achievement and the future they had hoped for. There is evidence that there are things that can be done to manage the condition, improve and, in some cases, recover. But key to coping with it all are relationships with the people around you – friends, family, colleagues and partners.

THE DIFFERENT LEVELS OF CFS/ME: MILD, MODERATE AND SEVERE

The levels of illness severity used in this book are taken from medically recognised British definitions (NICE 2007), and you may be surprised to learn that someone who is only considered to be mildly affected by CFS/ME can be living a very restricted life by usual standards. This is partly due to the fact that severely affected patients can be completely housebound and require 24-hour care. This wide spectrum of illness is very controversial and some people do not believe that these extremes can be part of the same condition. At the time of writing, expert opinion characterises the illness as a collection of symptoms that vary between sufferers and – as you will see from the contributors in this book – people can move between levels of severity at different stages.

Mild

People with mild CFS/ME are mobile, can look after themselves and do light household jobs, but with some difficulty. Most are working, continuing with education or sustaining the caring role they had before they became ill, but often at cost to the rest of their life, with restricted social, physical and leisure activities. They may need regular time off sick and have to use evenings and weekends to rest in order to keep going. Symptoms may include: aching muscles, breathlessness and exhaustion after low levels of activity, generally feeling unwell and heightened anxiety.

Moderate

Mobility is reduced and daily life is greatly restricted, with sufferers usually unable to sustain work or the life they had before they became ill. Levels of symptoms and mobility are changeable. Sleep is poor and disturbed, and, in order to function, they need a lot of rest and often sleep during the day. Other symptoms may include: muscle aches, joint pain, memory and concentration problems, palpitations, and a general flu-like feeling.

Severe

The severely affected sufferer may be able to carry out basic tasks such as face washing and cleaning teeth. They may need a wheelchair to get around and be unable to leave home very often, if at all, and usually have severe prolonged after-effects from any small exertion. They may be in bed for the majority of the time. They are likely to have severe difficulties with some mental processes such as concentrating. Other symptoms include: low tolerance of noise and bright light, severe pain and difficulty eating or talking.

Note to severely affected people and their loved ones

This book is written with a clear understanding that some of the advice and support presented will be frustrating for the 25 per cent of sufferers with severe CFS/ME. I completely acknowledge that for these people and their loved ones, seeing it as the same condition as someone with mild CFS/ME can be difficult as they are unable to participate in many of the activities discussed. However, medical thinking understands CFS/ME as a condition with different levels of severity that patients can move between. For example, from moderate to severe or from severe down to milder symptoms. The experiences of the contributors to this book show that movement between the severity levels is common. This book therefore covers all types of situations, so the majority of it will be most relevant to the 75 per cent who are diagnosed with mild or moderate CFS/ME. I hope that the loved ones of people who have the illness severely will find some support and understanding in the explanations contained and advice given.

THE WHOLE PERSON: CFS/ME, THE BODY AND THE MIND

It is important for loved ones of people with CFS/ME to understand that while the illness is a very real and debilitating physical condition, it also has a deep impact on mental well-being. Being able to talk about and manage the emotional side of the illness is vital as this can help sufferers cope and reduce additional difficulties that can arise such as anxiety and depression. This is also important in understanding and managing some of the physical symptoms, which can be made worse by stress and anxiety that are emotionally, and consequently physically, draining.

In order to stabilise symptoms, improve and even recover, it is important for people to think about the *whole* of their health, to try and balance an awareness of symptoms, activity, rest, relaxation as well as looking after their mental state and emotions. Neglecting any of these areas, or letting any of them dominate, makes coping much harder. For example, someone with CFS/ME who feels overwhelmed by fear, and continues to live at the same pace as they have always done, will find that ignoring the physical signals of their body will lead to increased symptoms. This does not mean that they are to blame for the illness, but that the condition is extremely frightening and hard to cope with. Another person may react to being so ill by becoming focused on a particular symptom, spending a lot of their time worrying about it and scanning their body for evidence of it. While this is understandable, it can also lead to greater anxiety and losing touch with the positive things in their life. Taking complete rest because of a fear of the meaning of symptoms is also dangerous as it can lead to further de-conditioning of the muscles, which actually makes symptoms worse.

Just as there are differences between the symptoms each sufferer experiences, so there will be many differences in how they cope with having CFS/ME. Our personal preferences come from many factors including personality, previous experience, current life stage, responsibilities and beliefs. It is important that the people around a sufferer can keep supporting them to work out what is right for them as an individual at each stage of their illness, because this can be very changeable and vary at different points. This book can help you to do that by offering a variety of ideas that reflect the diversity of people with CFS/ME and their needs. Having an understanding of what the issues are will help you to relate to your loved one in a more natural way so that you can vary how you help to suit you both. Even when it is difficult to understand your loved one's CFS/ME, this book offers many ideas for valuable practical help that can be offered. This book is for all of you. I hope you can recognise yourself in its pages and find the support or advice you need.

CHAPTER 1

What is Chronic Fatigue Syndrome/ME?

THE DIFFERENT NAMES FOR CFS/ME

Chronic fatigue syndrome and myalgic encephalomyelitis (CFS/ME) are the most commonly used names for a complex condition that can affect people in many different ways, varying in symptoms and intensity during the illness. A syndrome is a collection of symptoms that can be experienced by people who have that condition and there are various different names that are used for illnesses that are believed to fall into the same group.

Myalgic encephalomyelitis or encephalopathy (ME)

This name was at one time believed to describe the illness but is now not considered to be medically accurate. Although 'myalgic' means muscle pain, and 'encephalomyelitis' refers to brain symptoms (i.e. difficulties with speech, memory and concentration), 'encephalomyelitis' actually means inflammation within the brain and spinal cord, and there is no evidence that this is present in people with the illness. However, the advantage of this name is that it does sound suitably serious.

Post-viral fatigue syndrome (PVFS)

Many people who get CFS/ME develop it following a viral infection so doctors sometimes use the name 'post-viral fatigue syndrome'. However, as yet there is no definitive evidence that a viral infection directly causes the condition, and in some people who get CFS/ME there is no evidence of a viral infection having been present.

Chronic fatigue syndrome (CFS)

A chronic illness is one that lasts over a long period of time and to get a diagnosis of CFS a patient will have had symptoms for six months or more. This name was first used because, unlike ME or PVFS, it does not assume a cause that has not been proved. All people with the condition have fatigue, but also many other symptoms so this name can feel very limited in its description of the illness, with many sufferers considering it to be inadequate and even insulting.

Chronic fatigue immune dysfunction syndrome (CFIDS)

This is the name most frequently used in the US and refers to changes found in the immune systems of some, but not all, sufferers.

Fibromyalgia

This is believed by some doctors to be on the same spectrum of illness as CFS/ME and it can have features that overlap: brain fog (see p.22 and p.109), pain, fatigue and sleep problems. Fibromyalgia means nerve pain and this can be a symptom in CFS/ME, but fibromyalgia is diagnosed when the predominant problem is chronic widespread pain. There are differences in triggers, needs and treatment for this diagnosis.

Why CFS/ME?

I have decided to refer to it as CFS/ME in this book as this is currently the most widely recognised medical term for the illness and how the majority of patient groups refer to it in the UK. I am in agreement with the many sufferers who say that none of the names show the complexity of the condition and that this can get in the way of other people understanding how serious and disabling it is. You might have assumed that something called 'chronic fatigue syndrome' just means that a person gets very tired, but for someone with the illness this misrepresentation can contribute to their problems, making people's understanding of their illness more difficult by over-simplifying it. However, until a better name is found it is known as CFS/ME.

It is estimated that between 0.2 per cent and 0.4 per cent of the UK population are affected by the condition, which would mean there could be 240,000 people with CFS/ME in the UK alone (Action for ME 2006). At least one million Americans are believed to have it. Studies from the US show that it affects females more than males; people of all ages, but especially the middle decades; is seen across all social classes, and seems to be more common in ethnic minority communities than in the white population. One in four sufferers are considered to have severe CFS/ME but the condition can be so damaging across the whole spectrum that 77 per cent of sufferers lose their jobs due to the illness (Action for ME 2006) and people who are only considered to be moderately affected can lose the ability to do things most people take for granted such as working, playing with their children, driving and socialising.

THE SYMPTOMS

The statistics showing the percentage of sufferers who experience each symptom are taken from research done by the UK charity Action for ME, who asked over 2000 people with the condition how it affected them (Action for ME 2006). As you will start to appreciate, the symptoms each person experiences are individual to them and can be variable.

Fatigue

Extreme tiredness or exhaustion is experienced by all sufferers of CFS/ME but at various levels at different stages and even day to day. The fatigue is not like being very tired after a busy day. It is all encompassing, making usually automatic actions an effort and even simple thinking and decision making very difficult. It exists every waking moment, is not relieved by rest or sleep and can be made worse by even low levels of activity.

Sleep problems

Sleep difficulties can be varied and are experienced to greater degrees the more severe the condition, as well as varying on different days. Sufferers may find that the quality of their sleep is more than usually affected by alcohol, worry and noise. Long-term sleep problems are very frustrating, affecting energy, relationships and functioning.

Shallow sleep

In CFS/ME sleep is not as deep as it should be, so even when a patient has slept for many hours they will wake feeling exhausted. They can find that they are more easily woken by noise from other people, or even by their own body's natural movement during the night. This is also thought to contribute to some of the other symptoms of the illness as the restorative function of sleep is not fully happening. Muscles only fully relax in the deepest phases of sleep, so can be tense all night causing pain the following day. The lack of enough deep sleep also contributes to concentration and memory problems.

Disrupted sleep

As above, sleep can be severely disrupted with waking several times during the night for short or long periods of time. The dozy, half-awake state that allows people without the illness to go to the toilet without fully waking up and return straight to sleep is not always present in CFS/ME as deep sleep is not experienced in the usual way. The psychological impact of having the illness, worry about money, the future, etc. all add to sleep difficulties, making the relaxation required to sleep even harder.

Sleeping in daytime and less at night

A mixed-up body clock (or circadian rhythm) has been seen in many CFS/ME patients, affecting other bodily functions such as appetite and digestion. Daytime sleeping affects the quality and quantity of night-time sleep, and a negative cycle of disrupted sleep can be established as someone with CFS/ME struggles to get enough rest. Night-time hunger may be experienced, as they are awake more, which can add to weight problems.

Nightmares

Some patients experience intense and recurring nightmares, some of which reflect the anxieties of having a chronic illness.

Pain, aching joints, muscle spasms, headache

Two thirds of the sufferers surveyed have pain on a 'constant or daily basis' (Action for ME 2006) and this can be specific to a particular area of the body, most commonly the legs, or all over the body. This pain can range from a niggling ache to extreme pain requiring medication. It can be muscular pain or feel like it is right inside the bones.

Brain fog, memory problems, concentration problems

One of the most frightening aspects of having CFS/ME is the cognitive problems that can be experienced. Imagine being a young, intelligent person who is suddenly unable to string a sentence together or remember what you have just read. Eighty-nine per cent of people in the survey said that they felt the illness affects their ability to learn new things, with cognitive problems affecting conversation, work, planning, leisure, decision making and relationships (Action for ME 2006).

Palpitations, dizziness, anxiety

Some of the symptoms of CFS/ME are physiologically similar to the fight or flight response due to higher than normal levels of adrenaline, and a crossover can occur between physical symptoms and anxiety. For example, palpitations and feeling light-headed, which then increase anxiety levels as the person worries about what might be causing them, in turn increasing symptoms.

Fluey feeling, malaise, sore throat, painful lymph nodes

These symptoms are experienced in CFS/ME when there is no viral infection or temperature present, and it can feel like having the flu. Patients can feel achy all over, go hot and cold, feel overwhelmed by the need to sleep, with a stuffy head and sore throat. Action for ME (2006), found that 55 per cent of sufferers experience a severe flu-like malaise. If an infection or a cold is present as well as the other symptoms, this needs treatment and possibly medical attention to tell the difference.

Sensitivity to light and noise

In severe CFS/ME a patient can find that even low levels of light can be unbearable, increasing other symptoms such as headaches and pain. Similarly, noise may be experienced as overwhelming with relatively low levels of noise seeming very loud. Both of these symptoms mean that normal levels of stimulation can be intolerable, even painful.

THE DIFFERENT STAGES OF CFS/ME

Having these symptoms can be overwhelming as they can affect your ability to stand, walk, think, work, read, talk, drive, or maintain relationships, in fact everything most people take for granted. CFS/ME can feel like it threatens your very existence. When someone is diagnosed with CFS/ME, although they may be relieved to know why they are feeling so awful, they are facing an uncertain future. At this time there is no way to predict who will recover and how the illness will progress in different patients. Some people make a full recovery, others recover to some extent, and two thirds of sufferers will experience symptoms for the rest of their life (Action for ME 2006). As mentioned in the introduction, in the UK the condition is categorised into three levels of severity (mild, moderate and severe), which can be useful for deciding on treatment options and for understanding levels of effects and symptoms. People with CFS/ME may find these labels frustrating because calling a condition that affects your ability to function normally in every way 'mild' can seem insulting, and for those who have it severely, the mild category can seem like a minor problem in comparison. In reality, having CFS/ME can often involve moving between these different levels as the following case study shows.

CASE STUDY: CAROL

Carol, 64, has had the illness across all its levels:

> I have had ME since 1979, following a viral infection. Severity has ranged over the years from being totally bedbound (initially, and following gynaecological surgery in 1989) for weeks on end, to 85 per cent of fitness and everything in between, fluctuating according to mental and physical activity. I am at present around 70 per cent fit, though of course with major limitations in energy levels and activities.

Following is a breakdown of the stages of the illness, from the initial suspicions it might be CFS/ME to diagnosis to relapse.

Suspected but undiagnosed

People who have been ill for some time with symptoms that fit with the criteria for CFS/ME can sometimes find that their GP either does not know much about the illness or in some cases does not believe that it exists. If your loved one is in this position, they have found out through their own research that how they are feeling may be CFS/ME, but it is undiagnosed. It is important that they get a second opinion and have all the tests required to exclude other possibilities. Experts believe that the earlier a diagnosis is found and advice and information given, the better the chance of recovery.

Sudden or gradual onset

CFS/ME can seem to occur suddenly with someone waking up one day unable to get out of bed, or can develop over a period of months as a person describes feeling 'not right', but not being sure why, and gradually deteriorating. Levels of activity can steadily decrease as the person struggles to cope with day-to-day activities.

Boom and bust fluctuating pattern of 'good' and 'bad' days

This is a common feature of the illness in its mild and moderate levels, and means that symptoms can appear to randomly come and go. It can mean waking up one day feeling terrible, and sometimes having 'good days' with more manageable symptoms. It is likely that a sufferer will do less on a day that they are feeling worse, and try to get as much as they can done when they are feeling better, which can then result in increased symptoms and needing more rest. People who are working and have CFS/ME often fall into this category, as they sacrifice social and home life in order to be able to meet the demands of working, and may sleep during the early evening and at weekends in order to keep going.

Stabilisation

This means that a patient is experiencing a steady level of symptoms, which can occur at every level of the illness. They may be having many symptoms and problems but they are not as erratic. This can occur after having the illness for a while and gradually working out ways of managing it. It may occur while following treatment regimes as this is the aim of some, such as pacing, and a side-effect of others, as they encourage a balance of activities and rest and positive management of available energy.

Relapse

This can refer either to someone who has the condition and feels that they have gone backwards into experiencing a higher level of symptoms, or someone who had recovered and was able to lead a more 'normal' life becoming ill with CFS/ME again.

Being disabled

The definition of a disabled person that is used in the UK to support rights under the Disability Discrimination Act of 1995/2005 is as follows: 'a physical or mental impairment which has a substantial and long-term adverse effect on his ability to carry out normal day-to-day activities'. This can be seen to apply to people across the whole spectrum of CFS/ME and it has sometimes been recognised by awarding disability benefits to people who have the condition and are still able to work, which gives you some idea about the extent of the effects it can have on daily life. Considering yourself to be disabled can be both a negative and a positive thing as it brings with it the stigma of being different and separate to society yet can also bring recognition of the seriousness of your experience and help you get the support that you need.

Being housebound

People who are severely ill with CFS/ME find that they have very restricted mobility, so while they might be able to move around their home, they are unable to go out. If they have a wheelchair this does not address all the difficulties involved as there are many factors that affect symptoms other than walking. Noise, light, busy places and decision making all add up to stimulation that can be unbearable and greatly increase fatigue and other symptoms.

Being bedbound

People with severe CFS/ME can sometimes be unable to move out of bed, speak or feed themselves, needing 24-hour care. The smallest exertion results in unbearable pain, and they often need to be in a quiet and darkened room to manage symptoms.

Hospitalisation

Occasionally someone with severe CFS/ME will go into hospital or a care home in order to have their basic need for food and hygiene met through tube feeding and catheterisation. This is rare, but shows the extreme effects the symptoms can have in some cases, preventing the most basic bodily functions.

Spontaneous recovery

Sometimes CFS/ME patients report sudden and spontaneous recovery. However, this is rare and it is more usual that recovery follows their making big changes, gradual rehabilitation or treatment.

Recovery

If your loved one has had CFS/ME and tells you that they are getting better and no longer have symptoms, it is important that you try not to expect them to return to how they were before they got ill. This is something that they need to decide. For sustained recovery it is important that the strategies they have used to manage their illness continue to be a part of their lifestyle to some extent to minimise the risk of relapse. As the process of the illness is not yet understood it is hard to explain why this might happen, but anecdotal evidence suggests that a return to excessively demanding lifestyles, or big life events (such as having children, bereavement and moving house) can make relapse more likely.

WHAT DOES IT FEEL LIKE TO HAVE CFS/ME?

Everyone with CFS/ME has fatigue but will tell you that the tiredness they experience is nothing like how they used to feel after a hard day's work. Common things people say to try and explain it are:

> 'It's a bone-crushing tiredness.'

> 'It's like walking through treacle.'

> 'I feel like I'm very old.'

> 'It's not tiredness but heaviness.'

> 'It's like having lead weights attached to your limbs.'

> 'It's like the worst jetlag ever.'

> 'There is no word in the English language for it.'

'Normal' fatigue or extreme tiredness is the feeling that you are too tired to do something, but you can still do it. The fatigue experienced in CFS/ME means that you either can't do it or that if you try it is a struggle, causing pain and resulting in malaise and increased symptoms that can last for days afterwards.

There's a world of difference between not wanting to do something and not physically being able to! (Jane, 33, who is severely affected by CFS/ME)

To try to begin to understand what it is like to live with CFS/ME, consider how the following can make you feel:

The flu

Remember not a bad cold but full-blown flu where you had to be looked after and could barely stand up. Shut your eyes and try to remember what it was like to suffer that aching, misery, foggy mind, complete lack of energy and weakness. Now imagine not knowing what is causing it and whether you will ever get better, and you have the beginning of understanding CFS/ME.

Jetlag

The kind that lasts for days and leaves you disorientated, shattered, unable to concentrate, light-headed, craving sugar and just wanting to sleep. Shut your eyes and remember how that felt, now pretend that you don't know what's wrong with you, or when it will stop. You now have some idea of CFS/ME.

A new baby

Long periods of disrupted or missed sleep mean you have experienced severe fatigue and will know the effect this can have on your ability to concentrate and function. Add to this not being able to do simple things and finding it difficult and painful to even hold your baby and you can begin to put the fatigue of CFS/ME into context.

Overdone exercise

This can cause muscle aches, exhaustion, soreness in 'places you never knew existed'. Now imagine feeling like this after walking for only two minutes and not knowing why. Imagine it lasting for days afterwards and you can start to understand why CFS/ME is so frightening.

Here are some examples of the ways people with CFS/ME find their life has changed:

- 'I have the will, but not the way.' This is a description you may have heard elderly people use to describe their frustration with an ageing body, and is fitting as CFS/ME can feel as though you have aged 50 or more years. Try to imagine having to sit down at every opportunity, feeling so weak you can't walk to the corner shop, being unable to open a jar, needing help from others to do the simplest tasks, becoming forgetful and being dependent on others for basic things.

- Having to choose between two routine tasks because of limited energy, for example, whether to stop and put petrol in the car, or drive straight to your destination and risk running out of petrol because you are not sure that you can manage to do both.

- Watching the world carry on without you from behind a window; seeing people going out to work, socialise and play, and not being able to take part.

- Suddenly realising that you are holding on to a lamp post or door frame while every fibre of your body is screaming 'I need to sit down', and having to resort to sitting on the ground.

- Mary, 48, has had CFS/ME varying between severe and moderate for over ten years: 'What I miss most from my previously hectic and active life are those "little victories", the many sense-of-achievement moments that are part and parcel of normal getting things done at work or at play.'

- Noticing for the first time how few bus stops have seats, and how there are not many places to sit down in shops and town centres.

- Imagine going to a place you've always dreamed of visiting and not being able to see the main attraction, theme park, museum or gallery because you can't even stand and queue long enough to get in because it hurts too much.

- Imagine going to a concert and not being able to stand up long enough to watch the band and ending up sitting down on a sticky floor looking at everyone else's legs.

The three-part theory of invisibility in CFS/ME

An excellent description of what it is like to have CFS/ME is given by Mary Stow in the following theory. Mary, 48, has had moderate to severe CFS/ME for ten years and is largely housebound. Her ideas communicate the distressing impact the condition has due to its lack of recognisable face. She says: 'This invisibility is fundamental to the way we are treated by friends, family, the medical profession, benefits assessors, social services, insurers, the media, politicians, etc.' She has found thinking about CFS/ME like this helpful in making sense of her illness and coping with its emotional impact.

The first invisibility

The fact that you cannot see any signs of the illness. Your loved one may look perfectly healthy, or they may look 'tired' but there are no purple spots or missing limbs. If someone has a broken leg you see the physical evidence of the seriousness of their situation, and the impact it has on their daily life, and can sympathise even if you have never experienced one. As humans, we need to rely on quick information to make sense of a complex world, and so often judge others by how they look automatically. In CFS/ME this has the effect of preventing understanding, and downplaying the gravity of the illness or disability for the sufferer, increasing the isolation and frustration experienced.

The second invisibility

The fact that unlike other 'invisible' illnesses so little is known about CFS/ME that it sometimes isn't taken that seriously. If someone you know suffers from better understood invisible illnesses such as diabetes, epilepsy or bi-polar disorder you'll have some idea of what that means. For example, the effects of diabetes are widely known, such as the risks to the eyesight and heart, and we have an understanding of the distress of having to inject yourself with insulin and how diabetes affects life expectancy. Stephen Fry is an outstandingly articulate advocate and champion of those who suffer from bi-polar disorder. But CFS/ME is only really widely known for its controversial nature, or for making people 'really tired'. There is no agreed scientific or medical explanation or consensus on the severity or even the nature of the symptoms of the illness.

The third invisibility

The fact that those who are most ill are literally invisible as they are probably lying in a darkened room! Marching on Parliament is and will remain completely out of the question for them! As a result not only do the public not see the suffering of those who most need help, but also the view of the illness in the public domain is created by people who are less severely affected. The label 'yuppie flu' might be largely gone, but as long as those whose lives are more mildly compromised are the ones whose voices are heard by the public, the perception will remain that CFS/ME is not that serious.

WHY HAS MY FRIEND/RELATIVE WITH CFS/ME NOT DISCUSSED THIS WITH ME?

You may be surprised by some of the symptoms and not every sufferer experiences all of them, but there can be many reasons why your loved one has not told you about the full extent of their illness. Knowing about these can help you to understand more about what it is like to have CFS/ME and how it can affect your relationship.

Not wanting to get upset

It can be a very distressing experience being so ill and talking about it can make people feel very emotional. They may not feel comfortable doing this and so avoid telling you just how bad it can get.

Difficulty explaining how they feel

CFS/ME is such a complex and overwhelming experience that it can be hard to put into words. To explain all about it takes a lot of precious energy. The illness can also directly affect a person's ability to organise and express their thoughts, sometimes making it hard to retrieve words from memory.

To protect you

People don't usually like to upset those they care about and so you may find your friend or family member plays down how bad they feel so that you don't worry as much about them.

Shame

People with CFS/ME sometimes feel that it must be their fault that they are ill. Also, some of the symptoms feel shameful, for example memory and concentration problems bring fears of 'losing your mind'. Being unable to do simple things like cook a meal, wash the car or have a normal conversation, can be very embarrassing, especially if the sufferer does not understand why they are experiencing those difficulties.

Jon, 28, had severe CFS/ME and shows how people with CFS/ME can avoid telling others about it:

> I didn't want to be labelled with the condition, so I didn't claim benefits and avoided the doctors for a couple of years after the initial onset of my illness. I wish that had been different, but it's difficult to think straight with the illness.

Stigma

CFS/ME is sometimes seen by some as 'not a real illness' and fear of being misunderstood and judged as weak, a malingerer or hypochondriac can lead to a person playing it down. It can change the way other people relate to you.

Unsympathetic responses of others

After a few people respond to the news with a trivialising comment like 'Oh, I get tired', it becomes harder to face telling new people about it.

Being used to some of the symptoms

After living with CFS/ME for a while, you can begin to forget what it is like to feel well, so some symptoms are tolerated. For example, it is common for a patient with CFS/ME to no longer remember what 'normal' tiredness feels like. The kind of relaxed exhaustion you get after a hard day shopping or walking, which is relieved with rest and a good night's sleep, does not occur in CFS/ME. Sufferers develop ways of functioning in spite of their symptoms that you may not realise, for example doing less at home.

Denial

For some people the experience of the illness is so at odds with their self-image that they are unable to admit to people close to them the effects it has and limitations it brings. They may be struggling to accept that they are seriously ill and not talking about it is one way of coping with the fears they have for the future.

Distraction

One way of coping with the feeling of being ill is for people to avoid focusing on the symptoms, spending their time with you talking about other things.

Fear of being judged

There are so many changes that the illness brings to what someone is able to do that it can be embarrassing for a sufferer to admit that they no longer feel like themselves. They may protect themselves from expected rejection or judgement by not admitting how ill they are.

Believing 'you shouldn't moan'

People sometimes think it is wrong to complain about difficulties, so while they may tell you they feel ill, to go into the complex details of the symptoms would feel self-indulgent.

Boredom

It can get very repetitive living with a chronic illness as it is on your mind most of the time and sometimes you just want this to stop. A side-effect of this is the thought that if you are boring yourself then others will also find it dull, so you try not to 'go on about it', thinking other people don't want to hear.

HOW IS IT DIAGNOSED?

One of the reasons CFS/ME is difficult to diagnose is because it can have similar symptoms to many other conditions such as rheumatoid arthritis and multiple sclerosis, and many health problems can result in extreme fatigue such as anaemia and diabetes. These need to be tested for before a diagnosis of CFS/ME can be considered and it is also essential to exclude treatable sleep disorders such as sleep apnoea. This is done using a combination of blood tests and assessment to make sure there are no infections or other conditions that could be causing the symptoms. There is currently no specific test for CFS/ME and it can take a long time to have all the tests required to rule out other conditions before a diagnosis of CFS/ME can be made.

CASE STUDY: VANESSA

Vanessa, 36, has had CFS/ME ranging from severe to mild and describes her journey to getting a diagnosis:

Before this illness took over my life, I knew that I wasn't well but I tried to carry on as normal and pretend that I was OK. I sometimes would even think that I was going mad. I didn't seek help at that point and that is my biggest regret...I was frightened of the reaction 'Oh you must be depressed' or 'you're suffering from stress'. I knew deep down that it was more than this. Doctors need education to be more sympathetic in their approach to this type of illness, and not jump to conclusions; they are all too ready to dish out pills. (I was offered anti-depressants so many times but did not take them.) Mentally, I went downhill fast, I just needed to know what was wrong with me. Even after a year when I was getting better, I still had not had a diagnosis. I had to go with the diagnosis of CFS to my GP and insist on seeing a specialist, which happened months later...too late to do any good or help with the physical and mental problems I'd had.

The criteria for diagnosis may vary slightly in other countries, but the criteria currently used in the UK to consider whether a patient has CFS/ME is taken from the NICE (2007, p.34) clinical guidelines, which state that the following must be present:

Fatigue with all of the following features:

- new or had a specific onset (not lifelong)

- persistent and/or recurrent

- unexplained by other conditions

- has resulted in a substantial reduction in activity level characterised by post-exertional malaise and/or fatigue (typically delayed, for example by at least 24 hours, with slow recovery over several days).

And one or more of the following symptoms:

- difficulty with sleeping – such as insomnia, hypersomnia, unrefreshing sleep, a disturbed sleep–wake cycle
- muscle and/or joint pain that is multi-site and without evidence of inflammation
- headaches
- painful lymph nodes without pathological enlargement
- sore throat
- cognitive dysfunction: such as difficulty thinking, inability to concentrate, impairment of short-term memory, and difficulties with word-finding, planning/organising thoughts and information processing
- physical or mental exertion makes symptoms worse
- general malaise or 'flu-like' symptoms
- dizziness and/or nausea
- palpitations in the absence of identified cardiac pathology.

Your loved one will currently be experiencing some of these symptoms, and may have had others at different stages of their illness. Symptoms can change day to day and a lot of the fear that sufferers experience comes from the fact that symptoms often seem to be random and can be extreme, causing the sufferer to suspect that they may actually have a life-threatening condition that has been missed by doctors, such as cancer or dementia. These are common fears in CFS/ME and show how distressing the symptoms can be and how awful the illness feels. If doctors have carried out the exclusion tests for other illnesses, a patient can be reassured that they don't have a life-threatening condition. However, it is quite common for people to seek further reassurance from their GP or consultant during their illness because the symptoms can be so bad that it is hard to believe that there is not a more sinister cause.

CASE STUDY: VANESSA

Vanessa, 36, was severely affected and is now partially recovered. She describes the early stages of becoming ill:

> When my illness started to take hold and interfere with work I went to the doctor's and the start of many tests began. My bowels were one of the main problems and eventually I could not take any food at all, I went from ten stone to seven. They think my illness was brought on by a stomach infection months prior. I suffered with palpitations constantly, my body ached, breathing was hard, I could not bear noise and vibrations, major panic attacks started. I was bedridden for three months. Over this period of hell, which lasted about six months, I had no reassurance from anyone. I had to live day by day not knowing what was wrong with me, I thought I was going to die.

It is important to consider how a diagnosis of CFS/ME might affect an individual's self-image and social role. This can be more of an issue depending on the life stage of the person when they become ill, where they are in their career or family life. The more established their social and financial situation, the harder it may be to make the changes that can help to manage the illness.

In the UK, there is still an expectation that men don't show emotions and admit vulnerability, and this can have big implications for a man with CFS/ME. He may have the role of 'head of the family', be the main wage earner and may take responsibility for any heavy work around the house, and driving the family around. CFS/ME brings physical limitations to all these tasks which can be hard to admit.

'David', 53, has had mild CFS/ME for three years and is still working full time, but has not told many people that he is ill.

> Emotionally I find this condition very hard. My reactions to stressful situations can be sensitive, adrenaline in my system causes anxiety and palpitations. I resent the restrictions in my lifestyle. I try to keep optimistic that I will improve but keeping a positive frame of mind can be difficult. Some days I have to work really hard to manage, I find it difficult to express my thoughts and feelings about this condition.

It is much more socially acceptable for women to seek support and have adaptations made to their working patterns such as going part time, which can be necessary for someone to sustain work or engage in treatments. However, for women who hold traditional caring roles within their families, similar issues apply as they also need to adapt, and in most cultures women still do the majority of childcare and domestic work, as well as caring for older relatives, which can be difficult to change.

'Fran', 35, who has moderate CFS/ME, says:

I wish people would ask me what I need, I've always been there for everyone but now I need help too. Even though I can hardly walk some people still only see me as a strong person who's there for them.

WHAT CAUSES CFS/ME?

At the time of writing this book, the causes of CFS/ME are not fully understood and, as you can see from the confusion over its name, more research is needed into the illness. There is not even agreement over what school of medicine it should be placed in, and different specialist services have been set up by neurologists, immunologists and even within schools of infectious diseases (to reassure you, it is not infectious!). Various possible triggers for the illness have been considered, but no one theory has been proved. This has led some experts to believe that CFS/ME may in fact be several conditions with different causes that have similar symptoms. Others think it may be one condition that has a variety of triggers and forms of severity. Consideration of the whole of a person's life, taking into account everything that can contribute to someone becoming ill, including things that can keep the illness going, and those which get in the way of recovery, is also important. It is believed by many experts who treat people with the condition that social circumstances, beliefs about the illness and how a person behaves in response to having it can influence their chances of recovery, which is an increasingly common way of working with a variety of physical health problems.

Viral infections

The majority of people with CFS/ME (75%) say that it started after they had been ill with a viral infection such as influenza or glandular fever (Action for ME 2006). Even if this is the trigger, the symptoms of CFS/ME continue when there is no evidence of infection left in the body. However, not everyone who develops CFS/ME had an identifiable viral infection before they became ill, and not everyone who gets these infections develops CFS/ME. So infection alone does not fully explain why someone gets it, or how it progresses.

Persistent stress

Stress (either long term or acute) and trauma have been considered in some cases to have triggered CFS/ME, and there are links to some of the physiological changes that have been found in the body in patients with the condition, for example, in the cortisol levels of the immune system. Some patients describe experiencing extreme life events before they became ill such as bereavement or long-term work-related stress. However, not everyone who experiences extreme stress goes on to develop CFS/ME, suggesting other factors play a part too.

Hospitalisation/enforced bed rest

Some people develop CFS/ME after illnesses as described above, or after an operation or other period of bed rest. One theory about why this may trigger the condition is that resting completely sees a fast deterioration in muscle function and stamina, and that a too quick return to normal activity levels before full fitness has been achieved can send the body into an unbalanced state.

Studies have found physical evidence of changes and similarities in patients with CFS/ME in many areas, leading to theories about the cause. However, at the time of writing there is not a complete medical agreement on this and these changes are not found in everyone who has the condition.

Immune system

Abnormalities are found in some patients' immune systems but the cause of this is not clear. Sleep disruption can affect the immune system, increasing the chances of catching colds and other infections, a problem which is reported by many sufferers.

Neurological system

CFS/ME is recognised by the World Health Organisation as a neurological condition, which relates to the changes seen in the nervous system that may contribute to many of the symptoms. Research has been carried out looking at the muscles of people with CFS/ME and changes have been found in the cell mitochondria (energy-producing cells). Other current thinking is that messages to the brain may be disrupted in some way, leading to the experience of weakness.

Cardiovascular system

Stamina levels are found to be much lower in people with CFS/ME, and this can result from the rest that is taken in response to the symptoms. Changes in the heart muscle and blood flow, while not dangerous, can contribute to dizziness and fatigue.

Circadian rhythms

The human body is regulated by a 'body clock' in the brain that keeps the systems functioning over a 24-hour cycle. This controls sleep patterns, feelings of alertness, memory, appetite, body temperature, hormone production and the immune system. There is some evidence that in people with CFS/ME there is disruption of control over the body's rhythms (Williams *et al.* 1996), especially sleep patterns, which could contribute to some of the symptoms – fatigue, muscle aches, concentration problems, headaches, low mood and bowel problems. This also explains why CFS/ME can feel very similar to jetlag. Illness and stress can both affect the body clock.

Hormonal changes

Lower than usual levels of cortisol are found in some patients, which can contribute to fatigue, decreased alertness and sensitivity to light and noise (Kings College London 2008).

Digestive system

Fifty per cent of people with CFS/ME experience digestive problems, ranging from mild diarrhoea to irritable bowel syndrome and some of these believe that gut infections triggered their illness (Action for ME 2006).

Psychological health

There are still some doctors who believe that CFS/ME does not really exist and is 'all in the mind' of the sufferer, or is just a physical expression of mental health problems. This view has now been rejected by the medical profession, and if your loved one has a doctor who takes this attitude it is important to seek a second opinion as there is strong evidence that getting help early on in the condition can increase the chance of making a full recovery. There is a risk that anyone who has a chronic illness will experience mental health difficulties because of it, such as anxiety and depression, and these may need to be treated as well.

Personality

There is evidence to show that people who develop CFS/ME are more likely to lead a very active life, pushing themselves to their physical limits, and have high standards (Houdenhove, Bruyninckx and Luyten 2006). This is not in itself the cause of the condition because not everyone who has these traits gets the illness, however, it does have interesting implications for how someone copes.

Genetics

There is evidence from twin studies that differences in certain genes in the immune and nervous system can be identified in patients with CFS/ME (Nye and Crawley 2007), showing a possible predisposition to the condition in how the body responds to environmental triggers such as infection, so that some people may be more likely to develop it than others.

Toxins

There are people who believe their CFS/ME was triggered by environmental factors such as toxic waste or mercury dental fillings. There is no scientific evidence for this.

These changes are not all considered to cause CFS/ME. Some are understood to be factors in maintaining symptoms once the person is ill, while others may make some people more likely than others to develop the illness. A whole person view of an illness is valuable in any physical health problem because it allows you to consider all the things that might affect how the illness developed, how best to manage and cope with it, and to help achieve the best possible quality of life. Another good example of this is diabetes, where genetics, diet, lifestyle and attitude to health all play a part in the development of the disease, and are vital to consider when living with the illness, and to help prevent further deterioration.

TREATMENT AND MANAGEMENT STRATEGIES

At this time there is no cure for CFS/ME. Treatments that are available have been developed from theories about what helps to manage symptoms and reverse changes that have occurred in the body. They all encourage management of limited energy and stamina through breaking down and spreading out activities and minimising overdoing it, to avoid increasing symptoms further.

Medication

There is no drug treatment that can cure CFS/ME but there are types of drugs that may be given to assist a patient to manage the symptoms. However, some of these have side-effects so careful consideration is required.

Sleeping tablets

May be prescribed for a short time to help manage a very difficult period of sleeplessness. However, these are not recommended for long-term use because they can be addictive and cause rebound symptoms such as depression, anxiety and sleep problems.

Anti-depressants

Some types of anti-depressant medications can reduce pain or have a relaxing effect that can help people with their sleep difficulties and help them manage anxiety. If your loved one has been prescribed one of these it does not necessarily mean that they have depression.

Pain relief

There are many types of pain medication that may be bought or prescribed depending on the type and severity of the pain.

Muscle relaxants

These may be given to reduce aches and pain.

Graded exercise therapy (GET)

Some studies have found good results for improvement, and even recovery, among mild and moderately affected people using GET (Powell *et al.* 2001). This is a physical programme of activity that uses exercise as the 'medicine', increasing the activity levels and aerobic exercise very slowly and by very small steps. The idea behind this is that the process of increasing physical strength and stamina reverses some of the changes in the body such as de-conditioning and can 'reset abnormal physiological pathways and thus reduce symptoms' (Nye and Crawley 2007). However, experts admit that the reasons for its effectiveness are not fully understood. This can be a difficult treatment to follow as it is slow, takes a lot of time and planning and ideally needs to be supervised by a suitably experienced therapist. It is important that the sufferer does not start exercising suddenly because it needs to be started at a low level or the symptoms may be increased. GET is looked at further in Chapter 3 if you are supporting a loved one who is following this treatment programme.

Cognitive behavioural therapy (CBT)

This is a psychological technique that is often used to help people with other physical health problems such as chronic pain, arthritis and cardiovascular disease. Offering this treatment does not mean CBT therapists believe CFS/ME is 'all in the mind', but it works with the links between physical problems, thought, emotion and behaviour to find ways of managing illnesses better. There is some evidence that this can help improve symptom management and quality of life of people who have CFS/ME.

For example, if you had a broken leg, and were told to rest and stay off the leg, there are different ways you might react:

- *Emotion*: you feel frustrated and angry that you cannot walk easily so you might have the following thought...

- *Thought*: 'I can't stand this, it's not fair, I'm going to go crazy stuck in the house for weeks', so you might choose the following behaviour...

- *Behaviour*: go out, walk about and stand on the leg without crutches.

- *Outcome*: increased pain and longer recovery time.

By looking at how the ways we feel, think and behave interact, you can see how the way you respond to having a physical problem such as a broken leg might increase its difficulty and impact. A different reaction to the same injury, working within the limits of the leg, would have an alternative outcome.

For example:

- *Emotion*: you feel frustrated that you can't do what you want to do but you think as follows...

- *Thought*: 'This is awful, but in a few weeks I will be back to normal.'

- *Behaviour*: rest the leg as advised to and do something you enjoy.

- *Outcome*: the leg heals as predicted.

Other psychological therapies

There is good evidence that other types of therapy and counselling can also be useful in helping a person cope with CFS/ME (Ward *et al.* 2008) and make the best use of management strategies that can result in improvement. Interpersonal psychotherapy, integrative therapy, person-centred counselling, psychodynamic counselling and mindfulness cognitive therapy, when delivered by experienced and qualified therapists with knowledge of CFS/ME, can assist the sufferer to consider their situation, their reactions to it, their relationships and support systems and strategies for coping. In the UK, many areas have counselling and therapy available on the NHS via referral by a GP. Where this is not available, private therapy can be found by contacting your local professional therapy or counselling organisation (see Resources section).

Pacing

Pacing is reported by many sufferers to be of use in managing CFS/ME, allowing a sufferer to make the most of their limited energy and learn to plan their daily life around their needs, in order to avoid overdoing it and increasing symptoms further. While the concept is simple, actually putting this into practice often means a huge shift in focus for someone who is used to always being busy. Learning to adjust to operating from within what can be very limited boundaries is frustrating, and can be depressing, so having support and understanding to do this is invaluable. Pacing is also central to GET and CBT treatments and Chapter 3 offers more information on these issues and how you can help a loved one who is following any of the strategies and programmes mentioned here.

CONCLUSION

By now you will have a better understanding of CFS/ME, what is done to treat it, what it is like to have it and why it can affect everything a sufferer does. In the next chapter we go on to look at what it might be like for you as a friend or family member of someone who has CFS/ME, and offer suggestions for what you can do to cope with difficult issues that might arise.

CHAPTER 2

CFS/ME and You (the Friend or Family Member)

The complexity, uncertainty, unpredictability and frustration of CFS/ME that the sufferer experiences are mirrored to some extent in the way it affects the people around them. You will find, depending on the relationship you have with your friend or family member, that you will experience some strong emotions and changes throughout their illness. This can be painful and difficult, and we will look at different ways of dealing with how it affects you and your relationship with them. It can be a very new and confusing situation and this chapter aims to help you make sense of this and help you find ways to cope.

Ian, 32, whose sister had CFS/ME, found it hard to relate to her situation:

> The main difficulty has been struggling to understand the cause of the illness and the lack of knowledge about it. It is difficult to

empathise with a condition without having experienced it, and I felt pretty helpless when discussing it.

YOUR REACTION TO THE NEWS

Following is a list of possible reactions and emotions to the news a loved one has CFS/ME. You may experience some of these emotions while the explanations of the other emotions may help when trying to understand the people around you. It is important to remember that whatever you feel, whether positive or uncomfortable, it is your natural reaction and it is what you do as a result that will matter to your relationship with your loved one.

Shock

Maybe you hadn't realised they were ill, or had not been taking them too seriously when they told you there was something wrong. You might feel guilty if this is the case and you may find yourself wanting to avoid them. You might be shocked if you know someone else with the illness or have heard that it is rare to recover from it. Maintaining relationships becomes harder with CFS/ME for many reasons, so you could try to:

- Apologise if you need to, and move on to what you want to do next – your friendship will be better for it.

- Find out more information about CFS/ME to help you as well as asking your friend/family member how it affects them. By reading this book so far you have probably realised the condition is varied and complex so don't just rely on general information to form opinions about the illness.

Guilt

Sometimes people feel that it is their fault that their loved one is ill, that they have put too much pressure on them in the past or have not done enough for them. Although stress is a factor in the illness, there is no clearly understood cause and it is not possible for one person to be responsible for another's whole situation in life. Things you can do include:

- Learn more about CFS/ME to help you understand that it is not your fault.

- Try to make sense of why you feel guilty and how you can be different now your loved one is ill.

Sympathy/feeling sorry for them

You will be upset and concerned that they are ill and may want to express this. Be wary of what you say as sometimes a need to show that you are sympathetic can result in a misunderstanding. For example, saying: 'I know, it's awful, I get so tired myself' to try and be sympathetic can be heard by someone with CFS/ME as 'There's nothing seriously wrong with you, everyone gets tired, get on with it' and can put up a barrier between you as they feel their situation has been trivialised.

'Millie', 35, a close friend of a woman with moderate CFS/ME, says she's found it hard to find 'the balance between understanding and being patronising because this can be a fine line at times'.

Things you can do to overcome this include:

- Try to be aware of how difficult it is to understand how it feels to have CFS/ME.

- Look to your loved one for information rather than assuming things about how they feel and why.

Being dismissive

If your reaction to hearing that they have CFS/ME is to assume that this means they are just very tired, this can make your friend or relative feel you haven't listened to them, or that you don't take the illness seriously. As the symptoms and effects of the illness combine to make it harder to be assertive (fatigue, brain fog, anxiety, self-doubt and low self-esteem), it is harder to keep explaining the details and is sometimes easier to say nothing. The combination of both these things can lead to a friendship breaking down. Things you could do to overcome this are:

- Realise that they have a serious illness and that you will need to work quite hard to understand what it is like.

- Be honest with them and open up to the fact that you are struggling to see what CFS/ME means. This can lead to greater understanding because it gives your friend or family member the chance to explain.

Denial

In some cases the news that someone has CFS/ME can lead to a friend or family member seeming to have no reaction at all; changing the subject when it is mentioned; not asking how they are; looking uncomfortable; or even stopping contact with the sufferer altogether. Reasons for this include:

- They may find illness or emotion hard to handle.

- They may feel inadequate, helpless and too embarrassed to admit it.

- They may find seeing a loved one suffer too hard to cope with.

- They may be reminded of another situation from the past.

- They might have already been looking for an excuse to end the relationship.

- They might find the shift in balance in the relationship impossible to adapt to.

- They might believe the person is imagining the illness.

This is a very difficult situation to deal with as the sufferer may feel that the person doesn't care about them and has rejected them. If you are ignoring a problem it will be hard for it to be resolved. However, I hope this book is helping you to make sense of the illness. If you know someone else who is having this 'denial' reaction you may decide to talk to them about it, but ultimately they will have to feel ready to address it. If this kind of reaction is not addressed the hurt that results can be very hard to mend later.

Love/protectiveness

You may experience a strong sense of love for them and want to make them better. This is natural and you may find it upsetting because you will quickly realise that you can't do this. Things you could try include:

- Find a way to express your love and concern for them while you try to work out what you can do. Ask yourself and your friend or family member what you have done to help in the past that you could do again.

- Whether you tell them by writing them a card or letter, or show them by doing something practical, turning this feeling into an action will help you.

- If you find it difficult to cope with this emotion speak to someone else about it.

- Be wary of the feeling of wanting to protect them. This can lead to people trying to take over or smother a sufferer, which may not be what they want as it reinforces their sense of helplessness. It can also make their management of the illness more difficult as it is important that they keep active to some extent.

- Ask yourself who you are doing the helping for. If part of it is to make yourself feel better, or less guilty, be careful to keep asking them what they need too, as this situation can lead to resentment on both sides.

Ignorance

Thinking 'I know nothing about that, I don't know what to do/say' is easily fixed. Be aware of the impact of showing anxiety because you don't understand to your loved one as they may well be scared and may need reassurance. Try not to add your fear to theirs. However, assuming that you know all about the illness because you read about it in a magazine or heard a story about someone who has it can also be difficult. As you have probably realised already this far into the book, CFS/ME is a very complex illness and covers a vast range of symptoms and levels of disability. It is unlikely that your friend or family member will be the same as an experience printed in a magazine or heard about in a conversation. This ignorance of the complexity of the illness can bring a lot of negativity as many stories will be of the worst case scenarios as they are more memorable: 'Oh, I know a woman with that, she lost her job and can't go out any more'. This can be very distressing to someone who has just been diagnosed and is looking for support. The reality is that CFS/ME can be devastating, but it is important that a sufferer can find some hope and positivity to focus on, so telling them about the worst thing that can happen is not helpful.

- Ask them about their illness, or do some more reading about the topic. The fact you are reading this book is a positive step forward!

- Be aware about what you are saying and ask yourself whether it is really helpful to the person concerned.

- Remember that some people recover, and many others find ways to manage the illness that improve their quality of life. Keeping hope alive by focusing on this is very important.

Helplessness

Thinking 'I can't help them, I don't know what to say or do' is a very common reaction to seeing someone you love suffering. Maybe you usually help them out with problems and this time can't see a way to, or maybe they have always been there for you and so you are not used to offering them support. If so, the section on changes in relationships (pp.64–83) may help you to adjust. If you felt helpless on hearing they had CFS/ME:

- Try not to feel ashamed but tell yourself this is a natural reaction. It is what you do next that is important because sometimes this reaction leads to people withdrawing from the relationship or saying nothing.

- This feeling often comes from not understanding the illness, which you can change by doing some reading (see the Resources section at the back of the book).

- You might be feeling that you can't be how you'd like to be for them. If you withdraw it is easy for them to assume that it is because you don't care, because people with CFS/ME can feel very low in confidence and isolated. If you are honest that you would like to help but you don't know what to do, this will give you both the chance to work it out and keep your relationship strong. You may decide that you can't do more than keep in touch and ask them how they are and no more, but this is better than seeming to have forgotten them. Avoiding the issue is also damaging because it can feel that you are rejecting them, as CFS/ME will be a dominant part of their life.

Indifference

You may think it doesn't sound serious, and if this is the case reading this book has, it is hoped, helped you to understand the illness better. If you feel that it doesn't affect you, ask yourself why you are reading this book.

- If you are concerned enough about your friend or family member to want to learn more about their illness it has already had some impact on you. The reality of life is that relationships of any level are affected in some way when one person experiences a life-changing experience such as chronic illness.

Anger

This may seem irrational but anger is actually a common emotion when faced with a big change in life. It does not mean that you don't love them but that the news has affected you strongly and you may feel let down or scared that they won't be there for you anymore. Anger is linked closely to loss and feeling abandoned and can be a powerful emotion. Ways to overcome this include the following:

- Be clear about why you are angry and find a constructive way of coping with it. Directing anger at your loved one without understanding why you are angry can be damaging to your relationship.

- Asking yourself 'What am I scared of?' or talking it over with someone you are close to may help.

Frustration

You may feel very frustrated with the limitations that have been put on their life by the illness: that they can no longer do the things you did together; that they aren't able to be as spontaneous; or that doing things with them has become painfully slow and has to be led by how they are that day. This can be very difficult to accept, especially if you have known them for a long time and it is distressing to see them struggle.

'Millie', 35, says that she has 'had to reconsider certain activities and make changes' and advises: 'Try to be there for them and be understanding and not get frustrated, this can be hard.'

You should also:

- Be patient. It isn't easy but by being patient you will learn to accept and adapt to the changes in the person affected and the frustration will ease.

Loss

Feeling that the person you know has changed and that now they are ill things will be different between you can lead to strong feelings of loss. This may take effort to negotiate, but trying to do this rather than assuming you know how the future will be will help you to cope with your fears. CFS/ME is not a static condition and people do improve, so trying to work round the impact it has had is important. You should also:

- Try to keep in touch with the fact that they are still the person you love. Making an effort to talk about things other than the illness with them will help you to remember this.

Worry and anxiety

You will certainly be worried about what it will mean for your loved one and will have a lot of questions. Shirley, 62, says 'When our daughter told us she had CFS I was anxious because I knew that it is a debilitating condition and also possibly one from which you never recover, leaving you permanently disabled'. She advises that you try to 'be there for them and be prepared for them to have really bad days and be positive, even if you are feeling very worried yourself'.

Trying to take in the news that someone close to you is facing such a difficult future can lead to high levels of anxiety and feelings of helplessness. You may find that you are spending a lot of time worrying about them and that this is affecting you – causing you to be upset and anxious. Worry can interfere with your daily life and in some cases result in physical symptoms such as tension, sleeplessness and headaches.

- Talk your worries through with someone, a friend, doctor or even counsellor.

- Doing some research and learning about how accurate your fears are may help you and give you ideas about what you want to do. Unfortunately in CFS/ME there is no predictable path that the illness will take; so being preoccupied with how awful things could become or what your loved one has lost, while these things may be true, won't help you.

- Trying to shift your focus onto the whole reality of the current situation is difficult but can really help you to regain a balanced view of the situation. For example, look at the difference between these two ways of thinking about the same person:

1. 'This is terrible, my friend is only young and he can hardly walk, his life is over.'

2. 'My friend is really ill but he is still the person I have known for years. He might not be able to do some of the things he used to but I am going to support him to enjoy what he can.'

Another, more uncomfortable, cause of anxiety is often about what it will mean for you that your friend or family member is so ill. You may fear:

- that your relationship will end
- that you will have to do a lot for them
- that they won't be there for you anymore
- that they will change
- that you won't be able to cope with seeing them suffer.

Some, all, or none of the above might happen but again actively working with changes and being honest about how you are feeling can help. Also, deciding what you are going to do to support them can help you to reduce this anxiety because you can then say to yourself 'I'm doing what I can'. Taking positive action is a good way of reducing feelings of anxiety by taking control.

Relief

It is often a relief for the sufferer and their loved ones to get a diagnosis as they might have been very ill for a long period of time and fear the worst. Ian, 32, says:

> I knew my sister had been unwell, so in a way
> it was a relief to find out the actual cause of the
> symptoms.

People who receive the diagnosis often say they feel like this because it can end months or years of complete uncertainty and they are now able to begin to take some positive action to get help. This does not mean you are pleased that they have CFS/ME, but that you are relieved that they have found out what is wrong.

However, you may think that getting a diagnosis will mean they can get treatment and will recover but, as Ian quickly realised:

> [My sister] discovered there is very little known about CFS and therefore putting a name to it did not give any easy cure or solution.

Although CFS/ME is a serious life-changing condition it is not a terminal illness. Many sufferers feel so ill with extreme unexplained symptoms that they fear they have cancer or MS and to find out that they have CFS/ME – while there are no easy cures – can bring about the beginning of taking some control and learning to manage the symptoms.

Jealousy or resentment

You may find yourself getting upset that they are getting so much attention, especially if this is a big change in your family or group of friends. This is an uncomfortable emotion and difficult to understand rationally as it doesn't make sense to envy someone with a serious illness. Emotionally, however, it can be explained by asking yourself: what is it they have that you wish you had? Some of the possibilities could be:

- attention
- concern
- affirmations of people's love
- recognition that they are suffering

- a reduction in responsibility

- being off work

- people are taking their tiredness seriously when you are tired too

- they are getting extra support that you could do with yourself.

Whatever the reason for you feeling jealous, it is important that you make sense of this for yourself and try to address the reason for it. If you can find a way to understand what you need, you can try to get your needs met. It is easy to feel guilty for feeling jealous and this to then lead you to resent and avoid your loved one, causing you and them more discomfort.

Managing difficult emotions

Feeling what we think of as negative emotions can be difficult, and you may judge yourself to be a 'bad' person for it. You may find you feel guilty or anxious for feeling how you do, adding to all the other difficult emotions you are experiencing.

An alternative way of looking at it is to accept it as a fact that you have those feelings, and that there is a reason for it. Sometimes emotional reactions to events come from our childhood memories and can be irrational and feel overwhelming because of this. Any emotion has a message for us and the most difficult can offer important opportunities to learn and make things better.

Some things you can do to try to understand how you are feeling:

- If you have someone you trust to talk to it may help you to make sense of your feelings to say them out loud.

- Writing can help you to work things out. Get a blank piece of paper and write about your feelings as freely as you can, without planning or judgement. Looking back on what you have written can help you to get a clearer understanding of what is happening.

- Ask yourself if these feelings remind you how you felt in other situations in your life. This can shed a lot of light on difficult feelings as you might find that there are similarities with another emotionally powerful event or relationship that you hadn't realised.

- Draw a picture of how you feel. This can help you make sense of confusing emotions by freeing your mind.

- If you are really struggling you might decide to seek professional help. One of the benefits of this is that as a counsellor or therapist does not know the person concerned you may feel able to speak more freely. A good counsellor will not judge you but is trained to help you make sense of your emotions and work out ways to cope with them.

CHANGES IN YOUR RELATIONSHIP WITH THE SUFFERER

CFS/ME can have a major impact on the relationships between friends and family members. As it affects every area of the sufferer's life, the illness can also have strong effects, both practical and emotional, on those around them and communication can become more difficult. Yet relationships with friends and family are important to the well-being and happiness of all of us, and when you have CFS/ME they are a vital part of coping. Positive friendships and family relationships can greatly improve a sufferer's quality of life, and difficulties in relationships can sometimes make the situation harder to cope with. CFS/ME changes so much for the sufferer that it can feel like a barrier between you and everyone else. This section will look at some of the things that might help you as a friend or family member support and cope with the impact of the illness.

How CFS/ME can affect relationships

Keeping in touch is more difficult

Factors like low energy, overwhelming symptoms, problems with memory and concentration and less ability to do activities can all change a sufferer's way of interacting with others.

Can put emotional barriers up between people

The strong emotional reactions that both the sufferer and friend or family member experience can be difficult to cope with, sometimes leading to a breakdown in communication.

The balance of relationships can change

Roles that exist in relationships such as 'organiser', 'supporter', 'vulnerable one' or 'strong one' may well be affected by one person developing CFS/ME – this can be very confusing and difficult to adapt to.

Affects how social time can be spent

If the sufferer is no longer able to take part in the activity that they have previously shared, the friendship can feel a bit lost.

*Being ill can bring up old issues, particularly
in family relationships*

Childhood memories and difficulties about a person's role
in the family and how they are seen and expected to behave
by their relations can be seriously challenged as the sufferer
changes.

Expectations can become a problem

As above, the way that you have become used to your loved
one behaving may now not be fulfilled, causing anger,
resentment and confusion. This is a very important aspect
of the process of CFS/ME as it is vital that a sufferer is able
to think more about their own needs in order to manage the
illness.

Can lead to the end of some relationships

In some cases a combination of factors can feel impossible
to adapt to and a relationship will break down completely.
Jane, 33, severely affected, says:

> It's simple really. Friends can either try to
> understand and educate themselves or stay
> ignorant and lose contact. It's at times like this
> you find out who your true friends are!

However, there can also be positive outcomes within a
relationship:

*Can provide an opportunity for relationships
to become stronger and deeper*

The difficulties described can be an opportunity for people
to get to know and understand each other better.

Can become a chance for people to give something to a sufferer
Some people find that the support they offer is payback for
help that person has given them in the past, and can be an
opportunity to show how much they care.

Can lead to new relationships
Sometimes the sufferer finds having CFS/ME can mean that
new connections are made and people find new ways to
relate to someone they didn't know very well before.

The following examples show that the illness can challenge
close relationships.

May, 31, friend of a moderately affected sufferer, says:

> I think that we (still) have a good, strong
> friendship. The worst bits have been to do
> with my own frustrations. As I have seen her
> begin to get well again, I have occasionally got
> annoyed when she is still reluctant to do some
> things that she used to really enjoy for fear she
> wouldn't be able to do them... We've always
> been quite frank with each other though, so
> these things get discussed!

'Sam', 35, explains the impact the illness has had on her
relationship with her husband:

> My husband blames his reactions on finding it
> difficult to accept things. My limitations also
> impact upon his and our joint abilities to do
> activities. It also impacts upon his expectations
> of where he thought we would be at this point
> in life. He too has had to greatly lower his
> expectations because we were 'outdoor' types.
> I got ill so early on in married life.

BEING THE MAIN CARER

A person who provides the majority of the care for someone with CFS/ME will have more complex needs than other friends and family members, and may not recognise that they are in this role, seeing it as 'just what I do'. Sometimes the pressures on them may not be fully understood or acknowledged by others. The role of carer can be carried out by anyone close, whether it is spouse, parent, sibling, friend or even child, and can be done in a formal or informal way. A carer is anyone who provides unpaid care or support by looking after an ill or disabled family member, friend or partner. Many people may 'care' for the person, but the 'main carer' will be the person who provides the majority of that care. For example, a main carer for someone with:

- *mild CFS/ME* may have taken over some of their domestic jobs, may drive them around, go to medical appointments with them and provide emotional support

- *moderate CFS/ME* will have taken on a lot of the sufferer's domestic work, including cleaning and shopping and may provide intensive emotional support

- *severe CFS/ME* may provide 24-hour personal care, including feeding, toileting, running their home and communicating with others for them.

All the issues discussed in this book can be relevant if you are the main carer for someone with CFS/ME and your involvement will probably span many more areas than more distant friends and family.

Additional ways a carer's relationship is recognised are:

- They usually have a good understanding of their loved one's needs, including involvement in any medical treatment and appointments. Their role makes them an expert in their loved one's CFS/ME and they may act as advocate or intermediary between the sufferer and other friends, family members and professionals.

- Their own need for support is complex due to the level of care they provide and the impact this has on them. Their own health, both physical and mental, can be affected by the demands of their role, which can be stressful and exhausting, especially when they have other responsibilities and work.

- The Resources section includes many sources of useful information and support agencies specifically for carers.

PARTNER RELATIONSHIPS

CFS/ME can have extreme effects on this closest of relationships, in some cases feeling like it is falling apart, in others becoming a source of unexpected strength and support. Most will be somewhere in between and involve many complex issues that can be difficult to get through.

Challenges in understanding each other and staying close

Communication is always important in close relationships as it forms the basis of understanding, negotiation and intimacy. Even when communication has been clear and open, the challenge CFS/ME presents is great because both partners can experience fear and confusion that can get in the way of understanding. People who had previously been quite open emotionally may feel that they can't tell their loved one exactly how they feel, as they don't want to worry them. Those who have not found it easy to be open in the past can now find that the gap between them feels huge. There will probably be big changes in the focus of conversation in the relationship as the illness can dominate the life and thoughts of both as they try to cope with its effects.

Changes in roles

Roles in relationships evolve to manage the demands of day-to-day life and when one partner becomes ill with CFS/ME their capability to meet the demands of their usual roles will be affected. This can shake the foundations of a relationship, putting extra demands on the other partner and affecting how they see each other.

Money

The financial contribution the ill partner has made to the relationship will in most cases change through long-term sickness from work, or having to stop work and claim benefits. This will in turn affect the quality of life and freedom of the couple's life together – which may lead to resentment and arguments.

Work

Being unable to work also has a huge effect on self-esteem and ability to feel a sense of achievement and involvement in the world; and can lead to envy, guilt, and anger at being forced into a different role by illness. These may happen on both sides, as the well partner may feel envious of the partner who is not working: seeing them as having time and freedom from the stress of work. Frustrated partners may accuse the person with CFS/ME of laziness and ask them why they don't just do something, which has the effect of dismissing the seriousness of the illness and alienating the sufferer. In this situation it is vital that a partner learns something about the physical reality of the illness.

Parenting

This presents the biggest challenge to a couple even during times of good health. When CFS/ME affects one partner the balance in the demanding practical, physical and disciplining roles of parenting will change radically.

Domestic

The division of work around the home, whether housework, DIY or home maintenance needs to change if the person with CFS/ME used to take any part in these activities. It is very important to understand the limitations of your partner's stamina, as in CFS/ME 'overdoing' any activity by even a tiny amount can lead to increased suffering for days afterwards. In some cases getting outside help with some domestic jobs will help stop you becoming overloaded. But be aware that being unable to do what are seen as 'simple, easy' jobs is very difficult to accept, and your loved one may struggle to change how much they do, even if they are suffering because of it.

Intimate changes between lovers

CFS/ME can have big implications for couples, causing physical and emotional changes that affect how they interact with each other. Sex is a complex and emotive subject at any time in a relationship and when a chronic illness becomes an issue it can be a big challenge. Every sufferer's unique attitude to intimacy and how this interacts with their illness will be dependent on many factors. Some people may feel too unwell to make love, and symptoms of pain and fatigue can make taking an active role in sex difficult. On the other hand, if both partners wish to try new ways of being intimate, negotiating changes such as the use of different positions, techniques or roles to maintain sexual contact can help. The endorphins released during an orgasm can actually relieve some of the discomfort, and help the sufferer to relax and sleep better. Seeing sex as more than intercourse can help you to find different routes to intimacy, such as more sensual play. Body image is an important issue here as CFS/ME can bring changes in weight and body shape, affecting how the sufferer sees themselves and their attractiveness.

Time together

Social activities that couples share often involve stamina and mobility (for example, shopping, playing sport, going for walks, watching concerts), and these can all become difficult with the physical limitations the illness brings. Adapting to these changes means compromising what both people would like to be able to do. It is important for the partner to understand that it is not that their loved one doesn't want to do the things they have always enjoyed together, but that they either can't or find it much harder to do so. Finding new ways to spend time together, or doing usual activities more slowly with rest breaks built in can mean that time together can continue to be enjoyable.

Changes in emotional balance

When one partner becomes ill the balance of support in the relationship can change radically; the more emotionally dependent partner may find there is less support available for them, if the sufferer previously provided a lot of the stability in the relationship. You may need to find ways of being more supportive to keep communication open.

Change in relationship focus

Relationships are often built on shared goals and future plans and these can be put into question with the uncertainty of CFS/ME. One partner literally being unable to take part in projects that the couple have previously done together can make a stable relationship feel shaky. Expectations and ambitions may need to be put on hold or let go of completely if the relationship is to adapt to the illness.

CASE STUDY: 'SAM'

'Sam', 35, has been both moderately and severely affected by CFS/ME and her marriage has come close to ending as a result of difficulties of understanding, and the changes the illness has meant to the relationship. The problems she describes are not unusual and have made managing the condition harder for her, at times resulting in an increase in her symptoms. This account is from her perspective, and shows clearly the effect her husband's reactions have had on her. He has not had his say, but as a friend, partner or family member of a sufferer, you might recognise the frustration, confusion and fear that may lie behind his behaviour.

I wish my spouse would understand my limitations and believe me when I say I have hit my limit when out and about; and that doing more will overdo it with severe consequences. Such consequences are never seen by the other person when they are in work the next day, and I am struggling at home alone. They do not see you in bed, and too ill to talk on the phone. Pacing is fine in theory, until in practice your spouse says 'Can you just walk further, it is not that far to walk back to the car! You cannot sit down here, there is nowhere to sit, you cannot be so tired that you need to sit on the floor in a shopping centre!' In such situations, a refusal to take on board the limitations causes you to push through the fatigue. Pushing through it leads to me suffering severe symptoms, being totally in bed for three days, just to have a

Sunday afternoon out. Then this has an impact upon my ability to do the housework and care for myself. This can further impact on lack of understanding and severity of the setbacks. For example 'It's dusty' or 'Why is the washing up not done', or 'My ironing is building up'. Such things can be taken as being cruel and putting pressure on the ill person. That is the last thing you need when in an acute or relapse stage. I would then talk about having such a bad day, which is difficult to grasp and leads to the other person thinking that all you want to talk about is being ill and appointments.

BROTHERS AND SISTERS

CFS/ME can present big challenges to these relationships as we develop patterns in how we relate to our siblings during childhood. When we get together as adults these roles often stay fixed and conflicts and difficulties can develop. Brothers and sisters can struggle to see the sufferer as an ill person in need of support, especially if they are 'the strong one in the family', or a busy person who others go to for support. This is often reported by people with CFS/ME, and when positions are reversed others may not know how to support them. Alternatively, in some families the attention and support that the ill sibling receives may be resented. They may also feel angry about the strain and worry other members of the family are feeling, especially if they have elderly parents.

Addressing these issues is difficult and the sufferer may not feel well enough to do it and can feel resentful if their loved ones avoid the issue. In some cases this leads to distance between siblings and many unexpressed feelings can build up. Many of the issues discussed in this book regarding understanding and supporting someone with CFS/ME are relevant here, as in adulthood siblings are often friends, with the added bond of family that makes hurt deeper and harder to avoid. The main consideration is to accept that CFS/ME means that a sufferer's life is changed dramatically and that they need to be different during their illness and, if they recover, avoiding relapse involves maintaining some of these changes.

Paul, 29, brother of a moderately affected CFS/ME sufferer, says:

> I feel that our relationship has gradually improved, as my sister has become increasingly open and honest as to what she requires from other people, in terms of emotional support and flexibility (to aid her changes in lifestyle). This has in turn led to my discussing aspects of my life I may not have done previously, at least not as openly.

PARENTS

Being the parent of an adult child who becomes seriously ill is a confusing and difficult situation. People with CFS/ME most often become ill in their thirties and so parents sometimes find that their child moves back in with them as they are nearing retirement, either by choice or necessity if they are not able to get their care needs met elsewhere. In times of serious illness it can feel as if the person has regressed to childhood, feeling vulnerable and wanting to be looked after. This is rarely a simple thing as it involves losses on both sides. For the patient, independence and adult functioning; for the parent, some of their freedom and the belief that their caring days are behind them.

When the sufferer does not live with their parent(s), the impact of CFS/ME on their relationship can be huge as both sides try to negotiate the child's return to neediness and potential reliance. If they don't live nearby, providing support can be very difficult and may lead to anger, denial, frustration and a great deal of worry.

It is unlikely that a person with CFS/ME is completely honest with their parent about how they feel physically or emotionally as often they will feel the need to minimise their parents' worry as much as they can. A downside of this is that the parent won't have enough information to fully appreciate either how ill they are or how much support they need. Being proactive in learning about the illness through reading and asking about how they feel can help overcome this barrier.

On the other hand, in relationships where an adult child usually relies on their parent for a lot of emotional support, the parent may find the detail of the level of suffering they are told very difficult to handle – especially if the sufferer is open about extremes such as having suicidal thoughts. In this situation getting support, either from other family members, friends or even professionals, and sharing the pressure is vital.

Asking the question 'What would you like me to do for you?', and being honest about what time and support you have to give, can help avoid unspoken resentment and anger that can come from having fixed expectations of what help means, on both sides.

CHILDREN

Understanding and offering support to the children of a person with CFS/ME might be something other relatives need to have a part in as understanding and acknowledging the impact the illness can have on children is important. For younger children having a parent who is different to other kids' parents can be isolating and confusing. For older ones not having the same level of interactivity they see other parents give can be upsetting.

Being the child of someone with CFS/ME will be different for those who have always known them with the illness from those whose parent becomes ill for the first time. For the latter, loss and change may be difficult to adjust to as the physical reality of the condition is invisible and the sufferer 'protects' their child from knowing how much they are suffering.

Friends can help children to understand about the condition and its effects, to work out quick but effective ways of explaining it to others, and offer them the chance to talk about how they feel. Communicate to the children that their parent has an illness that makes doing everyday things more difficult. It is important for children to understand that it is not their fault and that their parent is not choosing to avoid activities they used to do together.

Other ways you can help include the following:

- Friends, aunts or uncles taking children out for the day will undoubtedly be appreciated by both the children and their parent(s).

- Other family members may need to step in and provide some practical and emotional support to help the sufferer cope, such as preparing meals, tidying up, bath time, helping with homework, ironing and so many other activities that go hand in hand with bringing up children and that put a serious strain on someone with CFS/ME. (See Chapter 4 for more practical ways of helping with daily life.)

FRIENDS

Friendships evolve over time and have to adapt to big life changes, such as becoming parents, career changes or moving away, in order to thrive. With CFS/ME, the uncertainty of the illness and the extreme effects it can have on a person's ability to take part in everyday activities present a big challenge to even the closest of friendships. The outcome of the experience can range from the friendship becoming deeper to it coming to an unpleasant end. Being a good friend means different things to different people, but the main thing for friends to do if their friend is diagnosed with CFS/ME is to actively take responsibility for maintaining the friendship. Adaptations will be necessary in communication, socialising and support. Expectations will be challenged and need to be kept open to discussion. Chapter 3 provides ways you can support your friend, and Chapter 4 offers some practical advice on how you can help with daily life.

However, if you find yourself really struggling to keep your friendship going it may be worth considering what the balance of the relationship was like before your friend got ill. Ask yourself 'Did they do a lot for me, was the friendship balanced or did one of us mainly give and the other take?' These are harsh questions but may help you to understand why CFS/ME is proving to be such a problem between you. When the sufferer has previously been the one that is there for their friends, is generous with their time and goes out of their way to look out for people, becoming ill with such a debilitating condition will mean huge changes to their ability to maintain their expected role in a friendship, as in other areas of life.

CASE STUDY: 'FRAN'

'Fran', 32, found a lot changed when she became ill:

> Having CFS/ME has changed most of my relationships, and it was painful to realise that some people don't care about me as much as I thought they did when

they weren't there for me. One of my closest friends just couldn't cope with me being vulnerable and she wasn't able to support me. I realised how unbalanced our friendship had been, I had always looked after her. I ended the friendship because I felt so let down. My relationship with my cousin has become stronger and deeper since I have been ill. She's been really honest about her feelings (sometimes of helplessness and ignorance), open to learning about the illness, and supportive. She has never stopped asking how I am, and has been able to adapt to the limitations that the illness has at times put on our relationship. She says that she hasn't done much, but she has really helped me by being able to accept my illness and still see me as the same person.

COLLEAGUES

Specialist CFS/ME physicians believe that for people who are working when they become ill, the support they receive from their workplace is central to their chances of recovery. If you are a colleague and/or friend of someone with CFS/ME who is still working, currently off sick or returning to work after illness, there are things that you can do to help that will benefit you, them and your team. If your colleague becomes ill with severe CFS/ME they won't be able to work at that stage in their illness. However, people can get better over time and they may return.

- Ask how it affects them. Don't assume you know – keep communicating about it.

- If you feel uneasy asking them about it, be honest about that, they may feel like that too. Saying so can get you talking.

- Do some research. Taking the time to understand what CFS/ME is shows support and will make it easier and quicker for you to understand them.

- Understand how the symptoms may affect a worker's stress responses. In CFS/ME a high anxiety state has a physiological basis as the sufferer's system produces more adrenaline than a well person so that the body can meet the daily demands placed on it. This also combines with the fear and uncertainty of having a serious illness and overall can mean that the sufferer seems more anxious and short-tempered than they have been in the past.

- Know that CFS/ME does not affect your intelligence but may mean new ways of doing things. Jacqui, 55, says:

  > I would like people not to rush into my office and rattle off something and expect me to give a quick answer, but allow me to take in what they have said, or better still, if they could just speak at a normal pace I would not feel stressed and would be able to give an answer quicker.

- Don't judge them on how they appear to be coping or how they look – *ask* how they are feeling. So much in CFS/ME is unseen and sufferers become very good at coping with quite extreme feelings of illness. This can all be going on when they 'look well'.

- Agree with your colleague how they want you to approach them about it. Ask them whether they think it affects your working relationship, and, if it does, what they want to do about it. Some people will prefer not to mention it; others will appreciate having an invitation to discuss difficulties.

- If you have concerns about the way they are working, it would be useful to discuss this with them. In many cases making small adjustments to the way they do their job can make it easier for them to cope. Remember, they are still the same person.

Supporting an employee who is a carer for someone with CFS/ME

If a colleague has a partner or close relative with CFS/ME, some understanding of the issues discussed here about flexibility, understanding the fluctuations, complexity and seriousness of the illness will be important. They may also just want someone to listen to them, share their worries and stresses, or they may just want to talk to someone else about something completely different and light-hearted.

Supporting someone with CFS/ME to return to work after sick leave

Employers' sickness policies sometimes allow for a four- to six-week period of phased or gradually increasing hours to help the returnee adjust to being back at work. This may be difficult for someone returning to work who still has CFS/ME symptoms, as it may be a shorter time than their stamina level will allow and often leads to further sick leave and ultimately giving up work. There are other ways to manage this transition that are more likely to support a sustainable return to work. Consider:

- a temporary reduced-hour contract for a longer period
- a permanent reduction in hours
- allowing the use of annual leave hours accrued during the sick leave to continue the phased return over a longer period

- phased return to full duties that extends beyond the initial period

- a change in role

- a combination of these options.

Once someone has returned from long-term sick they may feel pressure to 'be well' and avoid any further sickness. When managing or working with people with this illness, it is important to understand that other more common health problems such as colds, the flu and menstrual problems can multiply the symptoms of CFS/ME and be harder to tolerate. Also be careful to understand that not all illnesses a CFS/ME sufferer gets will be caused by their condition, and that stress is not the cause of their illness, but one factor that affects them. Developing an understanding of the following areas will be helpful:

- Understanding of the process of pacing. Managing the limited energy and stamina of CFS/ME requires careful balanced use of rest and activities split into smaller sections and spread out. This can often mean that the person is able to do the same task but will do it in a different way.

- Understanding of the process of recovery. If your colleague is following the graded exercise therapy treatment programme, educating yourself about what this means will be useful. Generally, someone in recovery from CFS/ME will be following the principles of gradually increasing all their activities over time – which can be a slow and frustrating process.

- Understanding of relapse prevention. Once someone has made a substantial recovery from CFS/ME they need to continue to use some of the strategies that have helped them to recover in order to stay well, making sure that life is a balance of activity and rest, and that they consider their own needs when making decisions. It is very important that the people around them remember they have been seriously ill, and don't expect them to go back to how they were before. This is because a return to a high-stress lifestyle greatly increases the chances of relapse.

See Chapter 3 for more information on all these issues.

COMMUNICATION

Why it can be easy to say the wrong thing

People with CFS/ME often find that the reactions and comments that other people make about their health can be very hurtful and increase their sense of isolation. Sometimes these things are said with the intention to hurt, but often they are meant to be supportive and are said with a lack of understanding. As a friend or family member, you may find that something you say does not get the response you expect. This section aims to let you know about some common misunderstandings that occur with CFS/ME so you can communicate better with your loved one.

*'I know how you feel, I get tired too' or 'We all get tired'
or 'Well, I've got children, so I know what that's like'*

Sometimes people say things like this when they have just heard the name chronic fatigue syndrome and know nothing about the condition. They genuinely don't realise that it is much more complicated and are trying to be sympathetic. Another reason is that they may be expressing their frustration that someone else has had their problems with energy taken seriously while they are struggling to cope with busy modern life.

'Fran', 33, whose CFS/ME led to her whole life changing, says:

> I saw a friend I hadn't seen for ages and told her I had been really ill with chronic fatigue syndrome. She said I should try having children then I would know what being tired was. I was so hurt that I've never spoken to her again.

As you have read earlier, CFS/ME is nothing like the tiredness many well people experience that can be caused by a busy lifestyle, poor diet, stress and sleep problems. The fatigue in CFS/ME is not relieved by rest. There are multiple other seriously disabling symptoms and, most importantly, CFS/ME stops you from doing important things – being tired only makes those things harder. If you find yourself saying something like this, you could ask them what they feel like and use it as a way to try and understand their situation better. Assuming you know how someone else feels can get in the way of actually understanding them – we are all different. An alternative would be: 'I know I get tired, but I don't know much about your illness. What is it like?'

'You're looking really well'

This is a common remark made to people with this condition and is usually an honest observation because people with this illness can look perfectly healthy with no outward signs of a problem. It is a polite social comment that is usually made with the intention of making someone feel good. The problem in saying it to someone with CFS/ME is that they are highly unlikely to be feeling well and this remark only highlights the lack of understanding other people have about the reality of their life. Looking good becomes a different priority for someone with CFS/ME as they have less energy to spend on getting ready and usually get a different perspective on what is really important in life. When you can't do the most basic things, having nice hair no longer seems so vital. Be aware of judging your friend on how they look because it is only if they start to recover that looking well may reflect how they feel physically. You could try asking them how they are getting on, this will let them decide whether to talk about how they feel.

'I think I've got that, I feel tired all the time' or
'I feel like that, what can I do about it?'

Immediately asking for the help of someone with a chronic illness without offering them any understanding and support can feel selfish and dismissive to the sufferer, but it does happen. It may be that the person who says things like this is more comfortable talking about themselves than asking about problems they don't know much about.

Carol, 64, who has moderate CFS/ME, says that she often feels friends and relations don't want to accept her illness and she is extremely frustrated that people don't understand:

> It seems women are the worst people to give you sympathy, as they are often competitive...
> I have had many people react with comments such as 'chronic fatigue, I've got that if you ask me'.

Of course occasionally someone who says this kind of thing may be suffering from CFS/ME and can actually identify with the symptoms of the sufferer, which may lead to a supportive conversation. But in most cases it is a badly thought out comment that fails to acknowledge how ill the person is, sending out the message that their situation is not important. You could say: 'I'd like to ask you about that sometime if that's OK.'

'Maybe you just need a break' or 'Have a rest then'

A suggestion like this can be said in ignorance of the condition or it may be that the speaker does not want to think about how ill the person is. Saying something like this comes across as dismissive and hurtful because if it was as easy as 'taking a break' then the sufferer *would* take a break and recover. Usually in CFS/ME resting is something that is enforced because they are unable to do many of the activities they used to do. However, it is not the relaxing rest you are thinking of. It can often involve sitting alone, suffering pain, headaches, flu-like symptoms and palpitations to name a few, and is certainly not relaxing or enjoyable. Instead, you could ask them what they need or what does help.

*'Have you tried this supplement?' or 'I read
about this amazing treatment…'*

Be aware that there are a lot of quick-fix cures for CFS/ME advertised, especially on the internet and, like the diet business, if there was one thing that really did work for everyone it would be widely known. Mary, 48, who has severe CFS/ME, explains how these can add to the frustration of the illness:

> The 'well-meaning' offering of miracle cures made me so angry and upset. Apart from the fact they almost certainly don't work, suggestions like that have the effect of inadvertently downplaying the gravity of the illness or disability for the sufferer.

If you genuinely believe something is worth looking into, be careful how you present it to your loved one as it is easy to offend. You could research the product first, the claims that are being made and whether they are backed up by any credible organisation or charity, and *then* subtly ask your friend or relative if they are interested.

*'You're lucky, I wish I was off work' or 'I'd love to be
able to sit at home all day' or 'That's nothing, I've got
two jobs, three kids and a house to keep going'*

It may seem odd but people do actually express envy at what they perceive to be the life of someone with moderate or severe CFS/ME: having nothing to do all day, not going to work, having people to help you round the house, etc. What they are saying is that they wish they had more help and free time, but what the person with CFS/ME will hear is 'You've got an easy life' and that they have failed to understand anything about the condition. The changes having this illness brings are not choices: they are necessities and cost the sufferer dearly in terms of damage to self-esteem, lost income, unsure place in the world and a great sense of loss of achievement. In some cases someone with CFS/ME may have had to leave a job that they did not like when they were too ill to continue, but this does not mean they would rather have a chronic illness. Most humans thrive on contributing to society through working in some way. Given the choice of a boring job or going through the hell that is CFS/ME, most people would choose the job. Instead, try saying that you sometimes wish for more time, but that it is terrible to have to be ill to get it.

*'I've been working all day, I think I
know what it's like to be tired'*

This statement is another example of competitive and envious thinking that can be said by a working partner of someone with CFS/ME who is struggling to understand why they can't do more, or a friend desperately in need of a holiday. This sort of talk can drive a wedge between people because it assumes that the speaker is just as badly off. Try to imagine watching everyone else going to work, socialising, enjoying life and not being able to take part. If you are relatively healthy you will have many more opportunities and choices than your friend or relative with CFS/ME, and it is important that you try to understand that no matter how hard your life is, with this illness quality of life is considerably reduced.

Saying nothing at all

Just as problematic as the previous statements is when someone never discusses their friend or family member's illness. This may be through ignorance, annoyance or being uncomfortable. However, saying nothing can be very similar to saying something that a person hears as insensitive or dismissive, as it will give the impression that you don't take their situation seriously. If you find yourself changing the subject when they are talking about being ill or if you never mention it when you talk to them, ask yourself why this is and try to imagine the same thing happening to you. If something life-changing was happening in your life and other people behaved as if everything was the same, how would you feel? Why not be honest and tell your friend or relative that you don't know what to say!

If you have said some of these things or have heard other people doing so, try to look at the situation from your loved one's point of view. This can help you get some perspective on why those comments inadvertently hurt your friend or relative. All the comments described above are frequently said to people with the condition – they have all been said to me! But remember, when you are seriously ill with CFS/ME you are less able to be assertive and argue your point due to the fatigue and cognitive problems the illness causes. Hearing things like this can leave a person feeling defeated and they may well not tell you how it has affected them, which can seriously damage your relationship.

What you can say

Asking your friend or family member directly what their symptoms are and how they feel shows you care and that you are taking their illness seriously. Remember that it can be very difficult to put into words what the symptoms feel like and some people may prefer not to talk about it. If you are worried you will upset them or that you will say the wrong thing, or not know what to say, it can be helpful to be honest about that, for example:

> 'I'm not very good at this sort of thing but ...'
> or 'You don't have to tell me if you don't want
> to, but I'd like to understand how you are.'

Having this kind of conversation can help you to bridge the gap that can open up when a loved one becomes ill. It will help you to understand more about them and be more able to support them and deal with your own reactions to their situation.

Some of the people who have contributed to this book point out the importance of how you ask. For example Carol, 64, who has had CFS/ME fluctuating between severe and moderate levels of disability for 29 years, says that:

> 'How are you feeling? Any better?' is a
> depressing question to be asked when you are
> seriously ill.

Vanessa, 36, who was also severely affected, says that she wishes people would 'avoid questions like "Are you all right?" and "How do you feel?", "What's wrong now then?"' She would prefer:

'Tell me what you want me to do' or 'What would you like me to say?' The patient will either tell you to go away, or shut up and don't speak! Or will for example ask just to hold a hand, just be there, have a hug, a cry or chat about anything else apart from what's in their world at that moment. These are the things we remember!

Common misunderstandings

There are many features of CFS/ME that can have strong and sometimes strange effects on the things a person can do, how they behave and how they feel. You may find that some of this information helps you to realise that in most cases the differences are not personal to you, but caused by the effects of the illness.

'He didn't ask me about my exam, he doesn't care about me anymore'

Does your loved one with CFS/ME forget when you are going on holiday, or what your new girlfriend is called when they used to know all about your life? Forgetting things you have told them recently and important information about your life does not mean that they don't care anymore. Memory and concentration problems are a symptom of the illness and also when someone is experiencing high levels of fatigue, any energy they do have will be used up managing basic information, which can leave no room for remembering about other people's lives. Try to bear this in mind if you feel hurt that they haven't asked you about something and just tell them about it. It may also be that positive things that are happening in other people's lives are painful for them to think about if they are not able to do them.

'She gets so annoyed with me, maybe she has had enough of me'
Irritability and anger can come from frustration at being so
ill, combined with the increased adrenaline in the system
that can lead to powerful outbursts of emotion, crying, panic
and even childlike tantrums. You may find this scary and
bewildering but it can be an expression of long-built-up and
complex emotions.

'Sam', 35, who has been severely and moderately ill
with CFS/ME, explains that it is usually people closest to
someone who will feel the full effects of this because they are
with them most often, and feel safest with them.

> How well we get on relates to how well
> or otherwise I have been. I know there is a
> certain level of fatigue where I can blow up. So
> whoever one lives with automatically gets that
> bad side of the ME patient. Any other family
> members or friends typically get the more
> sociable side on better days.

'Fred', 45, the partner of a sufferer who is moderately ill with
CFS/ME, admits that at times it is difficult to understand and
cope with the moods that she experiences:

> Sometimes the illness causes stresses and strains
> in the relationship. Her adrenaline levels shoot
> up when she hits physical limits to what she
> can do – with consequent stress, frustration,
> upset and anger. My response wasn't always to
> be as patient as I should have been because I
> felt the anger was directed at me.

It is important to try to understand the reasons for emotional
outbursts and to make sense of what is being said. If your
loved one is directly attacking you for not helping them
enough there may be an issue you need to sort out. However,
if they are saying they are upset about how they are feeling

or how their life is but in a loud or angry way, the fact you are there does not mean they blame you for it.

'I never hear from her anymore, not even on my birthday, our friendship is over'

As discussed above, memory problems can account for forgetting special occasions and, for CFS/ME sufferers, not keeping in touch as much is more likely to mean that they can't rather than they don't want to. You may find that your loved one seems to put their own needs first more than they used to. It does not mean they have become a horrible person; they just need to look after themselves better to cope with the illness. If they cancel an arrangement it probably does not mean they have something better to do or that they don't want to see you. Keep trying to find ways of keeping in touch – they will thank you for it.

'They have lost their spark, they are not the person I have always known'

Fatigue, pain and concentration problems all have a big effect on a person's ability to be assertive, make choices and feel enthusiastic. This does not necessarily mean they are depressed. It can be that the illness makes it harder for them to take part in things you take for granted such as lively conversation and social occasions. The way you communicate together may well need to change so that you can keep contact going.

'They are not there for me anymore, they have no sympathy for my problems'

Hearing about difficulties that you are having may not seem like much compared to what they are struggling to cope with. Problems are relative to what you have experienced in the past. People who have gone through extreme experiences like disasters and becoming disabled often say they see the world differently. You appreciate the small things in life more when you realise that life is not going to last forever. You also see how much energy can be wasted on trivial things, which can mean less tolerance for the daily complaining that some of us do about the weather and who said what to whom. Talk to your loved one about how you are feeling; consider telling them that you miss their advice. If you are still feeling unsupported you may need to find others who can help you because when you have CFS/ME there is much less energy available to give to other people.

'They have changed, we have nothing in common anymore'

You may be struggling to get on with them if your relationship was based on very specific interests such as sport or a hobby that they can no longer take part in. If you value their friendship and wish to keep it going you may both have to work hard to find new common ground or keep in touch in a shorter form such as text messages or cards.

If any of these things have happened to you and you find yourself hurt by them, step back from the situation and try to ask yourself whether it has happened because your friend is ill. If it is, then this might be a good time to reach out to them and find out if there is anything more you can do to help keep your relationship going.

SUPPORT FOR YOU (THE FRIEND OR FAMILY MEMBER)

Whether you are the main carer, a friend or a family member trying to help, you may find that you need support. In some cases you will want to talk directly to your loved one about how you are feeling, although this will depend on how close you are, how they are feeling at the time, and how comfortable you feel talking to them about difficult issues. However, some of the things you are feeling may not be appropriate to tell them about as you don't want to burden your loved one with your anxieties or it may be too difficult to talk openly about emotions. Thankfully there are other ways for you to get the help and support you need to cope with how you feel. In the Resources section there is a detailed list of UK and international support groups, charities, telephone lines, internet websites and forums, as well as books that you can turn to for help. Other support mechanisms include:

- Talking to other friends and family members. Your concerns and problems may well be shared by another friend or family member, so you could try talking them over to look for reassurance and ideas.

- Talking to other people who have a chronic illness, or a seriously ill relative. Sometimes it is only after you have spoken to someone who is in a similar situation that you begin to understand the isolation, fear and complexity that come with coping with serious debilitating conditions, for both the sufferer and those close to them. CFS/ME has things in common with a lot of other long-term conditions in its effect on all areas of life such as money difficulties, impact on relationships and isolation.

- Counselling. If you would like help adapting to the changes that your loved one's illness has brought about, then counselling may be a suitable option. In the UK many local health services offer free counselling after a referral is made by a doctor, although there may be a long waiting list in some areas. Private therapy can be found all over the world. To find suitably experienced and qualified therapists, contact one of the professional bodies listed in the Resources section. Some offer reduced rates for people on lower incomes and online therapy is a fast developing area, and can increase accessibility.

- Trying to ensure others take their turn in providing support for your loved one.

- Support groups exist in some areas for the friends and family of people with CFS/ME. Joining one and chatting in person or on an online forum to people in similar situations may help you cope with your situation better, gaining understanding and more ideas.

- Making sure you look after yourself too by eating well and getting enough sleep, as well as having plenty of breaks from caring for or worrying about your loved one. This will help you stay refreshed and make it easier for you to be there for them, giving the support they so desperately need.

- Moderate exercise such as brisk walking and swimming has proven benefits for relaxation, lifting mood, promoting deep sleep, stress management, and general well-being that can help maintain your physical strength and mental health.

- Developing something that is just for you, whether this is time alone relaxing, an exercise class, a hobby or time away visiting other people. This can actually help you to stay strong for your loved one, as well as making life easier for yourself.

See Chapter 3 (pp.149–152) for more ideas on looking after yourself.

CONCLUSION

In this chapter we have looked at how you might feel having a loved one with CFS/ME, why misunderstandings can occur, what you can do to deal with difficult emotions and how you can look after yourself while you are supporting them. In the next chapter we look at ways you can understand and support your loved one as they cope with CFS/ME.

CHAPTER 3

Supporting your Loved One to Cope with CFS/ME

As you have probably realised by now, CFS/ME is a complex illness with a wide range of physical, cognitive and psychological symptoms, as well as having a huge emotional impact on the sufferer and the people around them. This chapter aims to show you how you can help with the symptoms and the emotional effects of the illness, the treatments and management strategies available, as well as how you can help your loved one stay stable and prevent relapse.

It is important to remember that everyone is different and no two relationships work in the same way. While some of the advice given may be helpful to one person, if you or your loved one would not be comfortable with the suggestion made then it should be avoided. Pressurising yourself to be something you are not comfortable with will not help anyone: it is important to do what feels right for you and your relationship.

HELPING WITH THE PHYSICAL SYMPTOMS

As discussed in Chapter 1, there are varying degrees to which the following symptoms are experienced. Some patients have most of them, some will have a few that change at different times during their illness. It is best to ask your loved one about how they feel regularly because the condition is so variable. For some of the symptoms below there is medication and other symptom control measures that your loved one may be given by a therapist or doctor. In CFS/ME discovering what works for you is often a process of 'trial and error' as individuals can vary so much, so you could help them to consider their options and support them to try new things if they wish to, to find out what the benefits or difficulties may be.

Physical symptoms

Fatigue

For people with CFS/ME, the tiredness is overwhelming; for people only considered to be mildly affected the most straightforward exertion can be a huge struggle.

'David', 53, who has mild CFS/ME, says:

> I would like people to know that the condition is very real. On a physical level I have managed to continue to work, but have little energy, and I have to think about every task, knowing that the consequences of 'overdoing it' can be physical symptoms of aches, pains, palpitations and feelings of exhaustion.

For people moderately affected having a shower can mean needing to rest for half an hour afterwards before you have the energy to get dressed. In severe CFS/ME, the effects can result in being unable to mobilise yourself enough even to walk to the toilet or brush your teeth.

How you can help

- Try to understand what they are going through and adjust your expectations of what they can do.

- Appreciate the difficulty they have with tasks you might consider small and look for ways you can help or take away the burden.

- Talk to them to find out which tasks are the hardest and how you can help them.

- Ensure you respect their need for frequent rests, patience and quietness.

Pain and aching

This is a frequently experienced symptom of this illness, ranging from mild aching, which can be irritating, to severe pain that requires medication to manage. There are many different types of pain experienced: muscle pain, nerve pain, joint pain and headaches. There can seem to be no pattern to the pain: sometimes it is in one place, at other times it is all over the body. At times it feels like it is right inside the bones, which can be extremely frightening, and understandably make the sufferer worry that they have cancer or another life-threatening illness. If someone who already has chronic pain caused by conditions such as spinal problems or arthritis gets CFS/ME, they may have difficulty getting a diagnosis and engaging in treatments. As the muscle aches and pain in CFS/ME do not come from injury or disease, it can be difficult to make sense of what they can do without increasing other pains they have. They may start avoiding doing any physical activity, but that can make the symptoms of CFS/ME worse. It is important that treatment is given for each condition and that these take the other problems into account.

How you can help

- Try to understand what your family member is experiencing. Ask them about the pain and if there is anything you can do to help. As this symptom is such a large part of the condition, sufferers sometimes become so used to the pain that they may stop mentioning it, so it is important for you to keep asking.

- Practically, a hand, foot or shoulder massage can help to ease muscle aches and pains, and are also a good way of showing your affection. If you don't feel comfortable doing this you may want to pay for them to see a professional therapist as a gift. Be sure to ask your loved one how they are and what helps them as some types of pain experienced (e.g. nerve pain) can be made worse by touch.

- Headaches can be quite common. Noise and bright light can make them feel even worse, so allow your loved one to rest in a quiet, darkened room.

- Support them to have their medication reviewed if it is not working well.

Muscle spasms

Linked to the pain in CFS/ME, muscles can go stiff and won't work correctly. For example, hands can be affected, making writing, opening jars and doing up buttons difficult or even impossible. Legs can get very stiff if the patient sits still for long periods of time.

How you can help

- Try to help your friend or relative move around a bit to minimise the chances of stiffness.

- Massage and stroking can help relax and ease these symptoms to some extent.

- Help them to manage the fear this type of symptom can bring so they can change their thinking on bad days from 'My hands aren't working, I must have MS' to a more helpful 'My hands are playing up today, it is the CFS/ME and it's not always like this'.

Muscle weakness

This comes from a combination of other symptoms and the de-conditioning of muscles that results from being less active. This leads to a feeling of weakness that can make doing routine things such as washing the car and lifting even small boxes very difficult. People often find it difficult to admit this, so you may not be aware of this occurring in your friend or family member.

How you can help

- Be aware of changes in your family member's facial expressions or postures. This might help you to notice when they are finding difficulty with something but don't want to admit it.

- Find a way to alleviate the task in hand without taking over. Sharing might be useful by asking if they could do a 'lighter' task, while you attend to the 'heavier' task. This way your friend still feels they are contributing but not straining themselves too much.

• Encourage them to rest sitting up with their feet on the floor. Frequent resting in a lying position reduces physical stamina in a short period of time as the heart has less work to do.

• It is important that people with CFS/ME keep moving within the limits of their stamina, even if this just means walking around the house. This can help prevent further deterioration in muscle strength.

Palpitations/heart racing

This is a common symptom and can be very frightening as it can feel like you have a heart problem. If your friend experiences palpitations and they have been checked over by their GP to ensure there is no problem with their heart, there are other things you can do to help.

How you can help

• Reducing anxiety about this is very important. When they experience palpitations, talk to your friend calmly about what is happening and help them to tell themselves that this is a symptom of CFS/ME and is caused by excess adrenaline pumping around the body and nothing more sinister.

• Suggest your friend tries diaphragmatic breathing. Relaxation and breathing techniques can be helpful to reduce this symptom. Try going through the following technique with your friend. Imagine that there is a balloon in your stomach, place one hand on the chest and one on the stomach, and breathe deeply and evenly as though you are trying to inflate the balloon. Try to breathe deeply enough so that it is your stomach that moves the most. This technique offers many benefits, increasing the amount of oxygen taken in, relaxing the muscles and bringing you back into the present moment and away from the catastrophic thinking that can lead to panic. If your friend practises this daily, when they are not feeling so anxious, this type of breathing becomes easy to do on demand.

Sore throat/swollen glands/fluey feeling/general malaise

People with CFS/ME frequently experience a general ill feeling. This can be a combination of sore throat, going hot and cold, aching, feeling under the weather and, along with the fatigue, can become their everyday state. This is an awful situation to be in and feels very close to having influenza (the flu). People with CFS/ME can become so used to feeling this way that they may misinterpret the symptoms as a viral infection that needs treatment. Or the opposite of this happens, and people with CFS/ME do not seek medical attention when they do have a virus. It can sometimes be very hard to tell the difference.

How you can help

- Checking body temperature is a useful way of telling the difference. Viral infections raise the temperature to above normal which is usually defined as 98.6 degrees Fahrenheit (F) or 37 degrees Celsius (C).

- Help them to develop kindness to themselves by acknowledging how awful it is to live with these symptoms. Once they have checked for infection, support them by telling them that it is the CFS/ME making them feel like they do; this can help reduce the fear of other causes.

Dizziness

Some people experience dizzy or light-headed episodes, which can be frightening, especially when they occur in public places. This can take two forms: faintness, usually experienced when standing up, or a feeling that everything is spinning and off-balance.

How you can help

- Remember your first priority when your friend or family member has a dizzy spell is to ensure they are safe and sitting down. Try not to get embarrassed if this is in a public place; your friend or family member will be feeling even worse.

- Changing position slowly and steadily can help them feel better. Try to help them relax and breathe deeply.

- Work out the best way to do what they want to do, this may be to either get home or find somewhere more suitable to rest.

Nausea

Some people experience this very severely and it is very unpleasant. It can make mealtimes a problem, with the enjoyment of food and eating taken away and appetite reduced.

How you can help

- Root ginger taken grated in hot water as a tea or added to food can help to relieve this; if this does not help medication may be required.

- Help them to work out which foods make this problem worse and avoid them.

- Work on finding ways of eating that minimise the effects, for example avoiding big meals and eating little and often instead.

- Helping them to notice what increases the problem can be useful to work out ways of reducing it, for example some people will find that moving quickly will bring on a surge of nausea so you could support them to move more gently when they are feeling like this.

- Some people with CFS/ME have symptoms of irritable bowel syndrome linked to this symptom, see p.157 for more on this problem.

Sensitivity to light and sound

This can be a problem for people with moderate and severe CFS/ME.

How you can help

- Encourage your friend to rest in a darkened and quiet room, while ensuring that other people in the house are respectful of their need for peace and dark.

- Consider using lamp light (rather than the main bright ceiling lights), turn music and television down or off, and keep voices lowered.

Carol, 64, who has had CFS/ME across all its levels of severity over the past 30 years says that she benefits from people allowing her the 'ability to crash out in isolation and total silence for as long as I need, whenever I need it'.

Sleep problems

The disruption of the sleep/wake cycle is a common feature of CFS/ME and can happen in many different ways, from sleeping a lot but waking unrefreshed, to sleeping very little. Establishing a good sleep routine is essential in maximising available energy levels, minimising some of the symptoms and resetting the body clock. This can be the cornerstone of stabilising symptoms, and sometimes recovery from CFS/ME. If your loved one has problems with sleep, it might be useful for you to understand how they are affected. If you live with them or see them frequently, you may want to offer specific help with 'sleep hygiene', meaning encouraging good routines with the aim of improving sleep. You may benefit from these good habits too!

MILD CFS/ME

People mildly affected by CFS/ME may not have any obvious problems with their sleep, but it is likely that it is shallower and less restorative than normal.

How you can help

- Regular routines are important to maintain a good sleep pattern so respecting a sufferer's bedtime schedule when phoning or socialising with them can help.

- Be aware they may need to leave an event earlier than you would like in order to keep to a good sleep routine.

- Encourage them to wind down the day by relaxing close to bedtime, for example by reading or having a warm bath.

- Ensure as much as you can that the house is quiet at night with no disturbances.

- Avoid major discussions close to bedtime to assist relaxation.

- Encourage them to avoid cigarettes, alcohol and caffeine in the evening; they all affect the quality of sleep.

MODERATE CFS/ME

For moderately-affected people sleep is likely to be a major problem and they often have to sleep during the day. All the tips above are useful for them as well as the following.

How you can help

- Help them to establish a good bedtime routine. Going to bed and getting up at the same time every day can help regulate sleep patterns as well as improve the quality of sleep. This might be hard at first, especially if they have not slept well, but it will soon encourage a more stable pattern of sleep.

- Staying in bed in the morning and sleeping during the day will make the quality of night-time sleep worse. You can help them to reduce this, if they are keen to work on it, by encouraging them to do something else when they feel sleepy during the day. Moving about a bit or going for a short walk can actually wake you up and energise you a little, even if it is a slow five-minute walk around the block.

- Help them to keep a sleep diary, recording times they have slept, how they felt during the night and the next day. This can be useful to help spot patterns in sleep problems and so make positive changes.

SEVERE CFS/ME

People with severe CFS/ME experience extreme sleep problems and their other symptoms can make getting any relaxing rest impossible.

How you can help

- Keep the bedroom and house as quiet as possible when they are resting.

- At this level, sleep may need to be taken whenever possible, so be mindful of the severity of your loved one's illness and check if they want to rest regularly.

- Jane, 33, who has had severe CFS/ME, advises: 'Create a haven for the sufferer to retreat to. It's important for family to allow a sufferer rest time, so a comfortable, warm place with lots of cushions, CDs of relaxing music, candles and perhaps a blind to cut out bright light may be essential.'

HELPING WITH THE COGNITIVE SYMPTOMS

As well as the physical symptoms of CFS/ME, there are a wide range of symptoms that affect the functioning of the brain, which can be very distressing as well as difficult to make sense of. People sometimes believe that they are becoming senile so may need a lot of reassurance from friends and family that they aren't.

'Fran', 35, whose moderate CFS/ME brought frequent cognitive problems, says:

> It is like everything is a blur and that things that you know are in your memory are not accessible. Like reaching through fog for something you thought was there but coming back with an empty hand and not knowing why. At times you think you are losing your mind.

Cognitive symptoms

Brain fog

This is one of the most frightening symptoms as it involves difficulty with the most basic thought processes that the average person takes for granted, such as finding the right word to describe something, having a conversation, or making a simple decision.

How you can help

- Ask them what they find difficult so you will better understand when it is happening.

- Listen to how they deal with the problem. Do they make a joke of it or try to cover it up? By helping them to accept it as part of the illness you will not only help them come to terms with the condition but also reassure them that it is not part of another serious disease.

- Be patient when waiting for them to think or speak. Rushing them will only add to the pressure.

- If your friend needs to remember important information for or during appointments or meetings, help them make a list of questions in advance or, better still, go with them to the meeting.

- If they feel overwhelmed, stop what you are doing or talking about and help take the pressure off by taking a break.

Memory problems

Understanding that problems with the memory are a common symptom of CFS/ME can help you when your loved one is struggling with this distressing problem.

How you can help

- If you see them struggling with remembering something keep reminding them that memory difficulties are part of their illness. This may help to reduce the fear and frustration associated with this problematic symptom.

- Help them to remember things by writing important dates down or by using a calendar for birthdays, anniversaries, special occasions, appointments, etc. Ask them if they would appreciate reminders.

- You could help them to find methods of memory trigger that suit them, some ideas are: using sticky notes in places that they can be easily seen; helping them to make routines associating important tasks with other daily events, such as taking medication at mealtimes; and keeping a notebook or diary close at hand so they can write something down when they think of it.

- Most mobile phones can be programmed to remind you about important dates or commitments; maybe you could do this for them.

- Help them to reduce the guilt that can be associated with not being able to recall the things that are important to their loved ones by letting them know that you know it's a symptom of CFS/ME and that you know that they care.

Concentration problems

Difficulties focusing on a single task such as reading or following the plot of a film are characteristic of moderate and severe CFS/ME. It can fluctuate in severity at different times, usually linked to the level of fatigue that the sufferer is experiencing, robbing a person of simple relaxing pleasures. Do not assume that if your loved one is not working then they will be reading and watching TV. It is highly likely they will be struggling with these activities.

How you can help

- Be patient if they ask you to fill in the gaps in a news or television programme you are both watching.

- Make a list of your friend's favourite TV programmes and record episodes so that they can be watched when your friend feels up to it.

- Plan activities around the times of the day when they feel most alert.

- Help them to find new ways of enjoying the things they love, for example listening to books read out loud either by you or on CD; this can be done when they feel like it and can be easier than reading.

Serena describes the extreme cognitive difficulties that can suddenly overwhelm someone with severe CFS/ME, and advises you to:

> Learn to watch for 'The Fade', and understand that it can happen at any moment. We look generally OK, as usual, but will lose track of what we (or they) were saying, the upper spine begins to slump forward at least slightly, hands fall to the nearest resting place. We may or may not appear to be listening, but likely will have some trouble processing what we hear. This isn't hard to recognise once you know what to look for, and shouldn't be mistaken for lack of interest, unsociable behaviour, or a permanent change in abilities or status. When this happens, we need to be seated immediately, assisted with completing any business transactions that may be underway, and probably taken home. Be sure to ask first, but hold any detailed discussion for another time. Long-time sufferers are very familiar with its effects, but won't be up for much conversation until it has passed, this may be quick, or take a few days.

HELPING WITH THE EMOTIONAL EFFECTS

The emotional effects of having CFS/ME are complex, wide ranging, vary from person to person and can be even more hidden than the physical symptoms of the illness.

CASE STUDY: 'FRAN'

'Fran', 35, had moderate CFS/ME:

> Even though I had frequent pain, couldn't do much at all and felt like I had the flu a lot of the time, it was how I felt emotionally that was the hardest to cope with. I was so angry that this had happened to me, scared that I would lose everything I had worked so hard for, I felt like I was grieving a lot of the time for everything that I had lost and the prospect of my life coming to a complete standstill. I felt as vulnerable as a lost child and still do. I cried a lot and at least once a week would be overwhelmed by a mixture of feelings that led to an extreme desperation, sometimes I wanted to die so it would all stop.

Some emotional effects

Anxiety

This is a complex emotional and physical symptom. In CFS/ME feelings of stress and anxiety are partly caused by the fatigue and muscle de-conditioning from lower activity levels. This is because the body has to produce greater than usual levels of adrenaline in order to help the person keep going with limited energy and stamina. At the point when energy reserves run out, the body starts to 'run on adrenaline' in order to keep going, which can contribute to palpitations, breathlessness, tingling sensations, muscle tension and dizziness.

Anxieties about what is happening to their body, worries about money and the future, and fears about whether they will ever recover, all add to the already high level of adrenaline in the body. This can lead to a feeling of being on edge, stressed, irritable and overwhelmed, making sleep and concentration problems even worse.

How you can help

- Try to understand the complexity of the physical symptoms and the fears that come from having the condition.

- Reassure your friend and help them to learn more about the illness. The more they understand about CFS/ME and its symptoms, the less anxiety they will feel.

- Support them to get involved in relaxing activities – yoga, massage, relaxation tapes and meditation are all things you could do together and can be adapted to suit your loved one's abilities.

Panic

The combination of increased adrenaline, unpredictable symptoms and anxieties can lead to panic attacks: an extremely frightening physical experience during which the person can believe they are dying or may collapse. This process is linked to the 'fight or flight' mechanism, which is a natural process that was useful in prehistoric times where being prepared to defend the self against, or run from, wild animals was a regular and necessary part of life. Now the things that threaten us are more wide ranging, but we can respond in the same way physiologically to the fear of losing our job or our health.

The body automatically prepares to fight or flee the problem in many ways, including loosening the contents of the bowels (which can contribute to digestive problems); sending blood away from the brain to the limbs in order to prepare to run (which can contribute to dizziness); and producing more cortisol and adrenaline to power the effort (which raises the heart rate and can cause palpitations). All of these are symptoms in CFS/ME. If they are interpreted as being dangerous, which is understandable as they can feel extremely frightening, this can lead to a panic attack.

How you can help

- You can help by understanding the complexity of this condition, supporting them to minimise panic attacks and by having a plan of action in case one occurs, for example, by talking to them and understanding what the trigger is (e.g. shortness of breath, palpitations, feeling faint) and helping them to develop rational responses when they occur: 'This feels scary but it is just a symptom of the illness.'

- Try to avoid placing unnecessary stress and demands on them.

- Learn to read their emotions and whether they are having a good or difficult day.

- Panic attacks can become a pattern that is hard to break and may need professional help to change. See the Resources section for more about this.

- Be careful you don't support them to set up a cycle of panic by encouraging them to avoid situations in case they have a panic attack as this can reinforce their fears.

Grief and loss

It is important not to under-estimate the feelings of loss that someone with CFS/ME can experience. At the very least it means the loss of full health and mobility, but it can also involve losing a job, relationships, the ability to do things you love, as well as certainty, possibilities and hopes for the future. These can be experienced as a profound sense of grief, and bring overwhelming feelings of emotional pain and crying that can feel like a bereavement or broken heart.

How you can help

- It is important to be patient, understanding and accepting about the strength of how they feel, however hard this may be.

- They may benefit from some help to adjust to the changes and losses they have experienced by talking it through with a counsellor. These feelings can keep up during the illness because the uncertainty of not knowing whether you will ever recover makes reaching a point of acceptance of the situation very hard.

- Helping them to keep positive and hopeful for improvement by focusing on what they can do will help stop them becoming overwhelmed by grief. People can improve in time and become able to do the things they love again.

- When someone with CFS/ME loses a loved one, through bereavement or relationship breakdown, this may well have an impact on their physical condition. This is often under-estimated and it is important that the people close by are aware that on top of the pain of the normal grieving process, they may find their energy is further depleted and that their symptoms are worse for some time.

Anger, frustration and irritability

Anger often comes with unwanted changes in someone's life, and can be a very powerful emotion both for the person who is feeling it and the people around them. It can sometimes be hard to communicate or rationalise because it is so difficult to put into words, so instead comes out as irritability, snapping and getting annoyed about things that seem trivial. When you have a serious and debilitating illness like CFS/ME it is natural to be angry about how your life has changed. Being irritable also stems from the combination of feeling ill all the time, being worried about the future and a build-up of frustration. You may notice changes in your loved one's temperament and their speed of reaction to small things. Once again, it comes down to the anxiety they are experiencing, which can make them snappy and less tolerant of other people.

How you can help

- Help them to make sense of this emotion by letting them talk it through; this can assist you both to cope when they are really struggling. There will be something at the root of their irritable behaviour and talking is one of the best ways of finding out what it is and how you can help them deal with it.

- If this is not helping then professional help may be more appropriate.

- Realise that it is not you they are angry or annoyed with, it is the illness; understanding this will help you to take things less personally.

- Ask if there is anything you can do to help because sometimes isolation and lack of understanding can play a part in anger. It can be hard for them to ask for help.

Depression

This is far more than feeling low or sad. It is an overwhelming state where the sufferer's view of the self, the world and the future is bleak. They may feel despairing or numb, have lost hope and the ability to enjoy things. CFS/ME and depression have some overlapping features, for example fatigue and sleep problems, and one can get confused with the other. If they have had problems with anxiety or depression in the past (these are common problems that affect one in four of us at some time in life), these may return or be made worse by having to cope with serious illness. There is a danger that the physical reality of CFS/ME may be missed by medical professionals, or dismissed by their loved ones who assume the problem is psychological and that they can make it stop if they want to. Anxiety and depression undoubtedly make managing CFS/ME harder, but they do not cause it.

How you can help

- Notice how they talk about their life; are they feeling hopeless, useless or not feeling much at all? These can all be signs of depression and should be taken seriously.

- Tell the difference between symptoms of CFS/ME and depression. Saying that they can't do something is not the same as not wanting to do it. If your loved one says they aren't able to do something they used to do and they seem low about it be careful not to assume that it means they are depressed. People with CFS/ME are often unable to do things that might seem simple or easy to you because they physically can't. If they have also lost interest, however, they may be depressed.

- People can feel ashamed of having a mental health problem. Remind them that it is actually quite common. You could support your loved one to see the doctor and work out beforehand what they want to say, helping them to see that it is understandable that they could become depressed considering what they are coping with day to day.

- Any chronic illness brings an increased risk of becoming depressed and if this is the case for your loved one treatment may be appropriate with a counsellor, psychological therapist, CBT therapist and/or medication. Depression can be treated.

- Try to be patient and understanding. This is vital if they are struggling with such feelings and you may need to do some further reading about depression to help you cope with this (see Resources section).

- Take care of your own needs. Supporting someone with CFS/ME who is also depressed can be very hard work so make sure you have support too.

Trauma reactions

The experience of being seriously ill and the threat of losing everything that is important to you can be a very traumatic thing. Once someone with CFS/ME is improved or recovered they can have flashbacks and experience strong anxiety reactions if they have a feeling that reminds them of when they were very ill: for example, if their legs begin to ache or they see someone else struggling to walk. Underlying these experiences can be a deep fear of going back to the hardest time of their illness, and this is one of the ways the mind can try to protect us from further threat.

How you can help

- First, accept that what may seem to you to be over-reactions are actually a valid emotional reaction by your loved one. By accepting the severity of such reactions you will be able to make sense of your friend's feelings.

- Ask your friend or family member with CFS/ME if they are experiencing anything else that might make them think they are getting worse. This can help both of you to focus on the whole picture, reflecting on whether anything else has changed. It may help show that your friend is not getting ill again and is actually stronger overall.

- Give them a hug! They may just need a bit of reassurance that it is all going to be all right and the chance to talk over their fears.

Vanessa, 36, describes the emotional impact of becoming ill:

> I just wish diagnosis wasn't such a worryingly drawn out affair. The trauma of actually thinking I was dying made my symptoms much worse and my nerves are still recovering even now!

Suicidal thoughts

As we have seen, the experience of CFS/ME often means the loss of what is important in life: family relationships, friendships, work and colleagues, independence, hobbies and hopes for the future. This can understandably result in someone contemplating suicide and having 'intrusive thoughts' about death (when negative thoughts come into the mind even though we don't want to think about it). It is important to understand the difference between an *impulse* –

a fleeting thought – and the *intention* to act on such thoughts. If your loved one has told you that they are feeling like this it will be understandable for you to be worried.

How you can help

- If your loved one tells you that they are thinking like this it is important to take them seriously. At the very least they will be trying to communicate to you how bad they feel.

- Ask them if they think they will act on their thoughts or have any plans to carry them out, and this will help you to decide what to do. Having thoughts of wanting to harm yourself does not necessarily mean you will attempt suicide, but it is a good indication that someone is struggling to cope.

- Listening, believing and helping them to get support from a doctor or support group will reduce the chance of your loved one acting on such thoughts.

- It is also important to get support for yourself because you may find the worry has a big impact on your life. Share any feelings of responsibility by talking it through with other friends, family members, professionals or telephone helplines, taking care to respect your loved one's privacy.

- If your loved one is close to making an attempt on their life and they want help, you can take them to their doctor or local Accident and Emergency department (or Emergency Room) at a hospital for psychiatric support.

OTHER FACTORS THAT MAKE COPING WITH CFS/ME HARDER

There are many aspects of life that can affect the symptoms of CFS/ME, increasing them or setting someone back who has been stable or recovered. These things can also get in the way of using the strategies they find helpful to manage their condition. Taking this into account when these situations arise will be helpful.

Exacerbating factors

Common health problems

Of course people with CFS/ME get everyday illnesses just like anyone else. Catching the flu, a stomach bug or even a cold can bring a marked increase in their existing symptoms, and it can sometimes be hard to tell the difference. Some report a noticeably increased likelihood of picking up infections.

How you can help

- Try to be patient with the difficulties they are having. They probably feel a lot worse than someone who only has one minor illness to cope with.

- Help them to manage the distress feeling worse can bring by putting the increased symptoms into context: if they are caused by an infection, it will pass.

- Encourage them to seek medical help if they are experiencing symptoms that are new or much worse than they are used to. They may need medication.

- Consider staying away from them if you are ill; ask them if they would appreciate this.

- Understand that they may take longer than usual to recover.

Other chronic health problems

As is the case for any of us, some people who become ill with CFS/ME already have other serious and debilitating health problems, and some go on to develop them later. This can make coping with the condition even more complex and difficult, especially when the problem is a physical disability.

How you can help

- Try not to assume anything about their health; keep asking about it.

- Take other factors into account when you are supporting them. You may need to remind other friends, family and health professionals to do this too.

Heat

During very hot weather most of us will struggle with energy levels, sleeping and feeling comfortable. People with CFS/ME can find that their symptoms increase during a heat wave.

How you can help

- Support them to stay as cool as possible, especially at night; an electric fan can help with this.

- Ensure that they drink plenty of fluids.

- If nothing else has changed for them, remind them that the weather is probably the cause of them feeling worse rather than a setback. This can be important in reducing the anxiety that is felt when symptoms increase.

Menstrual periods

The female menstrual cycle can involve fluctuations in energy levels and emotional states in a well woman. With CFS/ME it can be that during the menstrual cycle the symptoms of the illness, especially fatigue and pain, can increase and be harder to cope with.

How you can help

- Be aware of the times of the month that they struggle the most and plan any activities carefully with them.

- Help them to acknowledge and manage additional physical and emotional difficulties and try not to take any outbursts personally.

Big life changes

The things in life that can be stressful for all of us, even when they are positive, can have an impact on the symptoms of someone with CFS/ME. Moving house, a new job or baby, bereavement, exams, financial difficulties and many other normal parts of life can make coping with the condition harder. This can be because they involve change in routine or physical exertion, or because they add to demands or anxiety levels which drain the energy.

How you can help

- When you are planning a change with your loved one be sure to discuss how you can take into account what helps them day to day. Can you incorporate pacing by breaking the process down into more manageable parts, for example?

- If a sudden event occurs ask them what they need to help them cope; this can get lost if everyone is affected and they may feel guilty about bringing it up.

- Consider whether whatever you are going to do should be an option at all. The costs to your loved one may outweigh the benefits.

- Taking their needs into account from the start will make life easier for everyone involved and can help you to avoid problems later on.

HELPING WITH MAKING POSITIVE CHANGES: TREATMENTS AND MANAGEMENT STRATEGIES

There are many things that someone with CFS/ME can do to help them cope with the condition; some suit some people better than others, and often this can only be discovered by trying them out. A lot of this will be about changing how they behave and think about things to help them to adapt to having CFS/ME. It is vital that each person has the chance to match their individual needs to treatments and strategies, and that these are delivered in a flexible way to meet those needs. We will look in detail at how you can help with this.

It is useful for you to appreciate why it can be hard for someone with CFS/ME to make changes, and follow medical advice or treatment programmes. You may find yourself wondering 'Why don't they just do what the doctor says?' or 'Why don't they just change?' Sometimes this is not easy, and understanding the reasons why will help you to support them and accept that they have to make changes at their own pace.

What can get in the way of making changes?

Being a 'doer' or having responsibility for others

People with CFS/ME are often busy and active people who others look to for support. They may well be a carer for other people, such as children or other ill relatives. Being able to use some of the strategies that can be helpful in managing the symptoms means that the person has to change their role and focus and make themselves more of a priority, which can be difficult to do.

How you can help

- Look at what you could do differently to help them with this.

- A common problem for people with CFS/ME is a lack of assertiveness when it comes to their own needs. Try to encourage them to tell people what they need and make time for themselves.

- If they are responsible for others (children or ill relatives) and they have to continue with these commitments, look at how you can help them. Can you share or take away some of the responsibility? Can roles be redefined within the household or family? Are there any options for doing things differently? These are important questions for you and the rest of the family to consider if the person with CFS/ME is going to start getting the help they need.

The treatment or strategy does not fit with their usual way of doing things

Some of the strategies that can help manage symptoms need good planning skills and discipline and they may be used to being much more spontaneous.

How you can help

- If your loved one is struggling with this you may be able to help them structure their days.

- Ask them if they want you to remind them to have regular rests and carry out other strategies they are trying to use.

- You could point out the things you notice that seem to help them manage and things that seem to make coping harder or make their symptoms worse.

Symptoms feel too overwhelming to make changes

Any new way of dealing with CFS/ME needs to be appropriate to the person's level of symptoms and stage of the condition. Feeling so completely ill can make it hard to see how anything small can possibly help, and it is true that some of the changes that do help can take a while to show positive effects. Not every strategy suits every person. A lack of motivation brought on by anxiety and depression can make it very difficult for someone to make changes. Mood swings and the inability to feel hopeful make positive action very difficult.

How you can help

- Accept that what works for one person isn't necessarily right for someone else. Everyone is an individual and finding the right treatment or management strategy can take time and patience.

- Deal with one issue at a time and help them consult a health practitioner to see if there are any suitable treatments for the anxiety or depression first. Once they are feeling more positive again and their motivation is improved, then move on to the more involved strategies for treating CFS/ME.

- Help them to find a strategy that is possible within their physical limitations.

Difficulty changing the habits of a lifetime/role fixedness

Often our routines and roles seem automatic and making changes even when we are not ill can be hard enough. To be able to really engage with some of these treatments a person needs to be able to put themselves first, and it may be the first time that they have ever done this.

How you can help

- Talk to them about how they see your relationship, your role as a supporter and invite them to say how they need things to be different.

- Have patience and help your friend slowly make the necessary changes. Too much too soon can be overwhelming to anyone, let alone someone with a chronic illness.

- Try to let go of how you expect them to behave and try putting them first.

Not wanting to draw attention to themselves/fear of ridicule

Many of the things that are helpful for sufferers of CFS/ME involve doing things in ways that are different to the way of modern life – slower, more simply and with less emphasis on achievement. This can be frustrating and confusing for others, and they or the sufferer can fear that it will be.

How you can help

- Support them to make positive changes by emphasising that their well-being is more important than what other people think.

- Try not to draw attention to how slowly your friend might be walking, for example, but instead focus on something else.

- Have patience and respect how they must be feeling. They will be well aware of how they have changed and may feel embarrassed or uncomfortable about it.

Not having enough support

Being isolated from friends and family can be a big barrier to engaging in strategies that can help with CFS/ME. If you have to run a home with very little support there is not likely to be much flexibility to begin new routines. If you have little emotional support it can be very difficult to cope with the fear and uncertainty that CFS/ME brings.

How you can help

- The fact that you are reading this book shows how much you care and how much you want to help, so it is to be hoped that your friend of relative shouldn't feel too isolated. Ask them if they feel that they have enough support and if there are any ways that others can help them.

- Work with other friends and family members to help out.

Other people not understanding

Others minimising the seriousness of the condition may make a sufferer's attempts to do things differently impossible. Lack of understanding of this illness is widespread and can lead to people being sidelined and judged, which will in turn make it harder for a sufferer to make changes that draw attention to their condition and limitations. Also, the strategies themselves are specific, slow and measured and so other people's need for someone to get back to normal or hurry up may put pressure on the sufferer that could actually harm their efforts. It is vital to remember that the only person who really knows how their body feels is the sufferer and they have to be in charge of any regime.

How you can help

- If you see this happening among family, social or work groups, help your friend or relative by challenging other people's misunderstandings or judgements. Before you do so, talk to your friend first to check that they want you to do this. Having someone who understands your symptoms and is willing to speak up on your behalf (especially when they don't feel assertive themselves), can be very reassuring and comforting.

Denial

Difficulty accepting the illness can be one of the biggest barriers to someone engaging in strategies that can help them. It is quite common in chronic illness for sufferers to be shocked that it has happened to them, and so protect themselves from the full implications of their condition by denying how bad it is. With CFS/ME this is made even harder by the relatively low level of support, understanding and knowledge that is available about the condition, which reinforces uncertainty. If your friend or relative does not fully accept that they are seriously ill, it is much harder to change routines and get help.

How you can help

- If you think your loved one may be struggling to accept their illness it might be helpful to ask them directly how it is affecting them and what kind of support they need.

- Give them time to come to terms with any diagnosis or acceptance of the illness. Be patient, but also keep reminding them that you are there for them to talk to about it whenever they are ready. Try not to avoid the subject.

Fighting CFS/ME

James, 35, describes a change in his relationship to CFS/ME that helped him:

> I learned that I needed to stop struggling in order to start recovery. I needed to go down before I could go up. This meant 'giving up the hope, but keeping the faith', i.e. stop actively hoping to get better (which provokes anxiety and stress), and simply trust that you will.

As James shows, the frustration of having big limitations, and a desperation to be better can actually get in the way of improvement. Struggling against the symptoms can increase adrenaline, tension and low mood, all of which get in the way of positive action. This does not mean they should give up: it means accepting where you are now and working with it, instead of against it.

How you can help

- Try to help your friend or relative to accept where they are and work with them to make the necessary changes to deal with the illness. Your acceptance of their current limitations and severity of their symptoms will help them with this.

Investment in staying ill

Sometimes long-term illness can bring positive gains along with its problems, for example getting support or being able to let go of some responsibilities. This can lead to a sufferer, or those close to them, not fully wanting them to recover. This is a difficult subject because it means that feelings that seem incompatible are felt at the same time. It does not mean that the person wants to have CFS/ME or that it is not real, but that there can be issues that block positive action.

How you can help

- These issues can be difficult so you may want to talk to someone else close to you to make sense of this before you bring it up with your loved one.

- Ask them how they would like their life to be different.

CASE STUDY: CHRISTINE

Christine shows how many of the above factors are issues for someone who realises that they need to do things differently for their own good, but find themselves struggling. It all comes down to accepting what they can manage at the moment and what they think other people expect of them. Sometimes it means finding new and different ways of doing things:

> I think that like me, most ME sufferers were 'doers'. One of the things I find most difficult is to say no to requests for help and to social events when I really, really want to say yes! Also it's difficult to have the courage or self-control to say 'I need to leave or stop what I am doing', when I find myself getting too fatigued. I don't like having to ask for special concessions. For example, I've just been on a weekend away but it was a full-on two-day event. I asked the organiser if I could just take part for two half days, rather than not go at all, and to my surprise, my wish was granted. So I had a lovely time and came home not too exhausted. But it took a lot of courage to ask for what I needed.

Recognising and understanding negative coping strategies

Like anyone in a difficult situation, people with CFS/ME sometimes try to manage difficult emotions and pain by doing things that are not good for them. If you think that your loved one is doing any of these be careful how you approach them about it – you risk being dismissed as not understanding how bad they are feeling. It is important that you do find a way to offer support in these situations, however, because they can make the symptoms of the condition worse, and can make depression more likely.

Drinking alcohol to excess

Alcohol is a depressant drug that may offer short-term release from problems, including pain relief. Although it can help you to get off to sleep, it actually increases sleep problems by disrupting deep sleep, and can lower mood, making developing positive coping strategies harder. Drinking becomes a problem when it is relied on to cope and there is difficulty facing things without it. Does your loved one drink every day, drink more than the recommended units per day, binge drink, drink in secret or drink during the daytime? Any of these may indicate a problem with alcohol. If you suspect your loved one is abusing alcohol it can be difficult to speak about this as it is a very sensitive area.

How you can help

- Get hold of some written information on the damage of alcohol from health centres and doctors and leave it in a place where your loved one can pick it up and read it.

- Tell them that you are worried about their drinking and ask if you can help them to cope with the illness an alternative way.

Comfort eating

Food is a powerful distraction, comforter and mood enhancer, but because people with CFS/ME are less active than they were, it is easy to put on weight, which can add to self-esteem, mobility and other health problems.

How you can help

- Be sensitive to this and maybe help them find other sources of pleasure to replace comfort eating.

- Suggest stocking cupboards with healthier foods and help them to find healthier alternatives, such as fruit, nuts and raw vegetables to replace some of their comfort foods.

- Notice when they use food to soothe themselves and give them the chance to talk about how they feel instead.

Using illegal drugs or over-using prescribed medication

Sometimes the desperation of illness means that people will try more extreme methods of relief which might not only be illegal but also risky for their health. Some pain medication can be addictive.

How you can help

- If you suspect your loved one is doing this, try to understand why and support them to have their medical care reviewed to find alternatives.

Self-harm

All the above examples can be seen as self-harm, and, in rare cases this can also include cutting or burning yourself which is done to relieve or distract from overwhelming negative emotions. If this is happening, it does not mean that they want to die. They will need sensitive support to find other ways of coping.

How you can help

- Talk to them and try to understand what is creating this behaviour. Try not to judge or be frightened by self-harm, but instead reassure your loved one that you are there for them and encourage them to adopt a different coping strategy.

- Support them by speaking to their doctor about getting them some emotional support.

Understanding and supporting your loved one to find out what works for them

The following techniques have all been found to be helpful for some people with CFS/ME. Some sufferers may be using one of them to help them cope; other people may use several strategies together and be working towards recovery. Graded exercise therapy, pacing and cognitive behavioural therapy all view CFS/ME as a physical condition and take a whole person view of treating it by encouraging a balance between activity and rest that suits each individual (NICE 2007; Powell *et al.* 2001). Ideally, the choice to follow a particular treatment regime or self-help strategy is made with specialist medical support, but unfortunately not all sufferers have access to this and may have to rely on their own research or the experiences and advice of others to make decisions. It is important to understand that not all approaches suit every level of illness or every person, and that the complexity of the condition can make some strategies impossible for some sufferers to use, so each person needs to choose what suits them and their experience of CFS/ME. Severely affected people can benefit from using parts of these strategies that fit in with their symptoms, especially pacing. Individually tailored activity management programmes for them are best delivered by medical professionals with specialist experience in working with CFS/ME.

Each individual's decision to follow a particular strategy or treatment must be respected as they know their symptoms best. Some of the theories and ideas are controversial; some are still being researched; and some may not be known to your friend at all. Be aware of this when you are talking to them. Further sources of information can be found in the Resources section of the book.

Pacing

This is a way of managing the limited energy available to people with CFS/ME through balancing activity and rest. This helps to break the 'boom and bust' cycle of overdone activity followed by increased symptoms that many sufferers find themselves in. There is a lot of evidence that this approach helps with the management of many physical health problems, including chronic pain, and Action for ME's surveys consistently find that over 90 per cent of their members benefit from using it (Action for ME 2007).

'Activity' includes mental effort and emotions, as well as physical exercise, because these also use up energy and can increase demands on the system. When pacing becomes a habit, people with CFS/ME can find that their symptoms stabilise, and even reduce, and their quality of life greatly improves. As a friend or family member of someone with CFS/ME, your understanding of how pacing works is valuable as it will help you to support your loved one in doing what is right for them. It will also help you to adjust your own expectations of them, which can reduce your frustration. Making new patterns of activity and habits for rest can actually result in being able to do more, with less upset, so it is worth everyone's effort to work together on this.

CASE STUDY: JAMES

James, 35, found that, for him:

> Pacing is key to recovery and, as a new tool, is something that your partner or parents can help you get to grips with and integrate into your daily life. For me, as a formerly highly active individual, the important thing was to structure the day around extensive rest periods (3 × 45 minutes). These were

periods for me to recharge batteries – to give myself the energy to continue for the next two to three hours. It also helped to think of my energy as a budget: where did I want to spend it and why? What activities 'cost' a lot and which were cheap? With my partner's help, I graded activities as needing low energy levels (e.g. meditating, reading), medium energy levels (e.g. washing up) or high energy levels (e.g. conversation). My partner and I divided up the day and week to ensure a balance, gradually changing that balance over time to increase the frequency or duration of high level activities. When designing a weekly framework, it made sense to think of specific goals: such as a five-minute walk once a week, building up to six minutes twice a week over a month. It also made sense to lower our sights, and – for once in my life – to play within my limits, rather than pushing them.

If you know the basic principles of pacing, you will be more able to support your loved one, or at least understand why they are doing things differently:

- Rest before you feel that you need to – this makes overdoing activity less likely.

- Plan rests before and after every activity or task – this helps the body to recover and manage energy more efficiently.

- Break activities down into smaller chunks – this helps gain a sense of achievement and makes overdoing it less likely, and the sufferer can actually get more done.

- Spread activities across the day and week – one of the aims is balance and stability, reducing and even avoiding the extremes of 'good' and 'bad' days.

- Plan ahead by thinking of the implications of every activity and decision – thinking about the smaller details may help you to anticipate problems and find ways around them.

- Pacing has a positive focus on improvement and recovery – a better sense of limitations is learned by using pacing and can lead to a person with CFS/ME increasing activity levels as and when they feel able from a more stable base.

Jane, 33, who has severe CFS/ME, states the importance of loved ones 'supporting them in maintaining a daily routine, for example, going to bed and rising at certain times, regular mealtimes, rest and activity times, etc.'

Graded exercise therapy

Graded exercise therapy (GET) is a demanding, slow and difficult treatment to follow but the benefits can be huge. The overall encouragement of structure, balanced routines of rest and activity, and focus on the self can produce a sense of control and progress that can empower the sufferer to gradually begin to achieve a stabilisation of symptoms, and so reduction in suffering. The 'exercise' is not the intensive aerobic kind you may do at the gym to begin with, and can include all physical activities that require stamina, including standing.

- CFS/ME is a seriously debilitating condition so the start level may be as little as a couple of seconds of movement for very ill people.

- Like sports training, it builds up gradually over time as strength and stamina increase.

- Levels are determined by how they feel after each activity. If it takes longer than ten minutes for the heart rate to return to normal and they feel worse, they have done too much.

- Rest is important for the body to adjust to the progress made, so rest periods before and after exercise sessions are important.

- It is very structured and needs to be taken as seriously as a job – taking priority over other things, with other activities fitted around it.

- The same principles can be applied to non-exercise activities to help build stamina and stay within manageable limits.

Cognitive behavioural therapy/psychological therapy/counselling
If your friend or family member is having one-to-one talking therapy to help with their condition, it is important that you understand that this does not mean they have a mental illness. Therapy can be helpful for addressing the impact of chronic illness, and working on developing coping strategies. Cognitive behavioural therapy is recommended for CFS/ME as it can be useful to help provide structure to encourage pacing, identify energy patterns, plan graded increases in activity levels and address some of the negative thinking traps that can result from having the condition. There is good evidence that other therapies can also be very beneficial and people with CFS/ME say that one of the most important things is that the therapist has a good knowledge of the condition and is able to integrate different therapies according to what the client needs (Ward *et al.* 2008).

CASE STUDY: JAMES

James, 35, had moderate to severe CFS/ME for three years, including several months confined to the house. He is now recovered and says:

> For an illness that appears to affect both body and mind (and to have both physical and psychological causes), it is unsurprising that there is unlikely to be a single treatment that sorts out the sufferer. More likely, it is worth trying a combination that is likely to be specific to the individual. For me, the key was understanding why I collapsed with ME/CFS. Was I the 'type' of person who would get ME/CFS and, if so, why? What aspects of my lifestyle were, for me, unhealthy? Psychotherapy really helped with this. I came to realise that I may have thought that I thrived on stress, but actually it was an anathema to my body, and I had actually spent much of my life trying to suppress chronic anxiety. Exploring the sources of the anxiety was enlightening, and understanding my psychological make-up liberating. Without it, I am sure that I would not have made progress. Cognitive behavioural therapy was also useful, particularly because it focused very much on practicalities of living with ME/CFS. But it could not penetrate to the psychological depths of psychotherapy; the two practices, for me at least, were not mutually exclusive.

Positive thinking

Having CFS/ME is hard to cope with and it is completely natural to feel low as a result. However, it is also easy to fall into patterns of thinking that are out of proportion to the reality of the situation, and these can make anxiety and depression more likely. Positive thinking is often discussed in self-help books or in therapy as being very important as it is linked to our sense of well-being and behaviour. However, it is a very sensitive issue to bring up with someone with a chronic illness as it can sometimes come across as insensitive to how the person with CFS/ME is feeling.

How you can help

- Noticing when your loved one is feeling low and defeated by CFS/ME can often be found in the language they use: 'Everything is hard', 'I can't do anything anymore'. You may be able to help them to manage any patterns of extreme thinking, but always acknowledge that they feel bad for a good reason or they could believe that their feelings are being dismissed.

- If everything is seen as completely negative ('My life is over', 'Everything is awful'), you could ask them if this is completely true and subtly help them to focus on the positive things in their life.

- If they are feeling a sense of worthlessness ('If I can't work I am worth nothing'), remind them of other things they can be proud of and recent accomplishments as well as the courage they are showing in coping with CFS/ME.

- If they are making unpleasant statements about themselves ('I'm useless'), remind them how great they are at other things and that it is the illness that is making them feel like this.

- You can help them to take a more balanced view of their life, strengths and positive relationships, especially if you know them well, by challenging negative statements they may make about themselves.

But be careful how you do this because it is important to acknowledge the distress they are experiencing. For example: 'I know you are feeling like there's nothing you can do at the moment but you are still the person I have always admired. I look at you coping with being so ill and I still see a strong/wonderful/lovely person.'

Alternative CFS/ME treatments

There are many non-orthodox treatments offered privately that make claims to treat or even cure CFS/ME. These can be very expensive and there is often no reliable research evidence for their effectiveness. Some people who have received these treatments describe them as amazing; others have found the same ones useless or even damaging. If your loved one is considering going for one of these treatments you can help them to evaluate the information that is available on the internet and in their literature, and check out the cost, qualifications, reputation and experience of the practitioners offering them. Someone who has had CFS/ME for a long time and already tried many things to try and get better can feel understandably desperate, which can lead to decisions that affect them financially, causing other difficulties. You could help them weigh up all the aspects of their choice and keep a balanced view of the possible outcomes.

How to help your loved one with these techniques

Whether your friend is following a programme of GET, using pacing strategies, having therapy or simply coping day to day with their symptoms, there are some really important things you can do to support them:

- *Help them to focus on progress* – because this is slow it can be very frustrating so it is important that other people help the sufferer to keep recognising how far they have come, even if it might seem like a small improvement to you, for example: being able to walk for two minutes without difficulty is 100 per cent longer than one minute.

- *Praise them by recognising their determination and focus* – understand and acknowledge what it takes to face the day with CFS/ME. The effort to keep a positive focus is something that can get lost in the struggle. You can act as a reminder.

- *Help them to plan their activities and rest* – structure and planning are key to using pacing and other strategies. You may be able to offer some organisational skills to help them.

- *Notice what happens when they try a new way of doing something and tell them what you see.* It can be helpful for someone else to act as a mirror so that the sufferer can see from another perspective how what they do and how they feel is related.

- *Help them make time for the things that they want to do* – making big changes in how you manage time can be difficult, and you might come up with ideas they hadn't thought of.

- *Encourage them to stick to their current level* – it is tempting for sufferers to push themselves further than they can comfortably go, and you may share their frustration and want quicker results. Try not to give in to this; more progress will be made overall if they take it gently because they are less likely to suffer a setback or major relapse.

- *Remind them to stick to their chosen strategies* – it is difficult to change lifelong habits and so people can slip back into old patterns of putting other people's needs before their own. You can help by noticing when they are not taking regular breaks or have stopped doing things that were helping.

- *Let go of any prejudices you may have about therapy* – if your loved one finds therapy helpful try to accept that, and discuss the revelations that emerge during the sessions with them if they want to. This can help reinforce change and will also help you understand them better. Going for therapy can take a great deal of courage and is often a challenging process, so expect that this might have its difficulties.

- *Understand that making changes is emotionally hard.* Your loved one will feel frustration, isolation and anger, because it is often impossible to see an end to the struggle. This can make engaging in any treatments hard and your support for this by acknowledging any difficulties can really help.

PREVENTING RELAPSE AND STAYING STABLE

If your friend or relative reaches stability with the illness or seems to have completely recovered, try not to forget they have been seriously ill with a condition that has affected them physically and emotionally. Forgetting the experience and impact of CFS/ME may lead you or others to place too many demands and expectations on them. It is important for a sufferer, and his or her loved ones, to keep the experience of the illness in the back of their mind. 'David', 53, advises being: 'sensitive, but not over-sensitive' to your loved one's needs and any changes that occur.

How you can help

• Ask them what they want and need and how they are feeling.

• Encourage them to continue using the strategies that helped them. Keeping the good habits of balance between activity and rest, and pacing themselves will make relapse less likely.

• If you are worried that they are doing too much, tell them.

James, 35, was severely ill with CFS/ME and is now recovered. He advises that:

> Partners, parents and friends still need to understand how stress continues to adversely affect me – and do what they can to avoid imposing additional stressors by having unrealistic expectations. They can also help by watching over me, pointing out any return to unhelpful behaviours (e.g. overworking).

• Understand that the experience of being seriously ill can leave its mark in the memory. Even though they may be physically better, emotionally situations that remind them of being severely restricted can trigger anxiety and distress that might not be rational, but are very real. For example, someone who was unable to stand for more than five minutes for years without pain may well feel anxious if they are queuing for a long time and their legs begin to ache. This is because their memory of that experience is closely linked to the sensation of tired legs and can bring up the strong fear that they felt at the time. This does reduce over time as they begin to trust their body again, and your patience, understanding and support will help.

- Help them to check out how real their fears of relapse are when they feel unwell by looking at the whole picture – their stamina, sleep pattern, balance of activity and rest and other possible causes for how they are feeling, for example: change, stress, or other health problems. This is often enough to help them to put how they feel into context, or if they conclude that they are becoming ill again, support them to make changes or seek help.

Understanding and supporting people with medical and treatment appointments

When you have CFS/ME there can be a big variation in what support is available according to where you live and, as we have seen, the types of problems that your loved one might seek help for. Some people will be receiving support from their GP, which may take the form of advice, monitoring and/or medication. In places that have no specialist service the GP Practice Nurse may be the main support. Some people with CFS/ME find that they don't meet the criteria for specialist treatment (which may be due to other physical conditions or level of severity); or they may decide that the available treatments are not for them. Specialist services offer a range of treatments, some of these are delivered in groups, and others on a one-to-one basis. It can be extremely distressing attending appointments as at these times the full implications of the illness are discussed which can be a very emotional thing, but the positive effects of seeing supportive professionals cannot be over-stated – feeling understood, experiencing a reduction in isolation, having an emotional outlet, a chance to ask questions and receive validation for how they feel.

How you can help

- Offer to drive them to their appointment, or help them to find someone else who can, well in advance. If they are having a bad day, not having to worry about getting there can make the difference between going and staying at home.

- If they are finding getting to appointments difficult for any reason (transport problems, feeling too ill, nervousness, being unsure about the treatment, etc.), encourage them to address the reason for this and call their therapist to try and sort it out. Services are often under pressure meaning that they have to discharge people who don't attend, which could mean the need for a re-referral, and then another long wait for your loved one.

- They may appreciate support attending the doctor and hospital appointments, and this can be helpful for you to understand what is happening.

- It can be useful to plan for some time available after the appointment to relax somewhere quiet to talk about what has been said.

- For the person with CFS/ME, having someone with you can be vital regarding brain fog and fatigue, combined with the stress of attending and difficulties concentrating. Having someone else listen to what is being said, take notes if necessary and even explain their symptoms and ask the right questions is a great help.

- If you are not able to attend with them you could help your loved one to make a list of the points that they want to cover before an appointment as this can be a very useful memory aid.

- You can also help pass on the information to other friends and family afterwards.

- It is also useful to remember that the physical and mental exertion of travelling to, waiting for and then concentrating on an appointment will take their toll on your loved one's symptoms. They may well find that they need to have nothing else planned for that day.

James, 35, advises:

> Help the sufferer by researching available professional options, arranging an appointment and sorting travel.

Jane, 33, who has severe CFS/ME, recommends:

> Look together carefully at the pros and cons of any treatment the sufferer is considering giving a go. Think about such things as how far they have to travel, as this in itself can be exhausting. What qualifications and previous experience of the condition does the practitioner have? What is the success rate from previous sufferers? What costs are involved? It might be worth setting any treatment a trial period of say three months and then reassessing the benefits. But ultimately try to support them in whatever decision they make.

OTHER THINGS THAT CAN HELP

The following are all things that people with CFS/ME have found helpful, and are also useful ideas for looking after yourself. They cover a wide range of ideas from different theories about how the body and mind work, which can be confusing so you may want to do some reading to help you choose something that suits you and your loved one. If you have an interest in any of them you could offer information on what's available locally, or you might choose to take part with them which can be an opportunity for you both to spend some positive time together. See the Resources section for more information.

Some ideas

Relaxation

Using recorded relaxations or visualisations, or deep breathing techniques such as diaphragmatic breathing (see pp.102–103) can help reduce tension and anxiety and make coping with the symptoms easier. Having a bath with luxurious products can also be extremely relaxing.

Meditation/mindful awareness

There is growing evidence that meditation can be very effective in helping people cope with chronic illness and pain, especially mindfulness meditation which helps you to live within and accept your current situation. Mindfulness, which is intentionally bringing awareness to the present moment in a non-judgemental way, has a powerful role to play in general health and healing for both physical illnesses, and depression and anxiety. Local Buddhist centres may offer short courses to help you with this and there are various meditation CDs and internet downloads available. See the Resources section.

Music

Music can be soothing, uplifting or a good way of relaxing and managing difficult emotions. You could make a CD of tunes you think your loved one would enjoy.

Massage/aromatherapy/reflexology

These can be very helpful for relaxation, pain management and overall well-being. If you can offer this yourself, do so, or you might want to buy them a voucher as a gift.

Alternative medicine

Some people have found that other therapies such as acupuncture, reiki and homeopathy have helped them. Although their effectiveness is debated within the medical profession, when provided by trained practitioners they can't do harm, and at the very least they offer the kind of care and individual attention that can be very therapeutic when you are ill.

Nutrition

This is an important part of energy management and self-care in CFS/ME and is covered in detail in Chapter 4.

Film and books

There is growing evidence that the arts can be a helpful tool for people who are ill to channel their emotions, and gain understanding of their feelings by witnessing those of others. Depending on what they feel able to do, you could lend them books or DVDs of stories you have found moving or life affirming.

Being creative

Similarly, painting, drawing, crafts and writing can all be a good outlet or distraction for coping with difficult times.

CONCLUSION

In this chapter we have looked at specific physical and emotional problems that can occur in CFS/ME, and how you can help support your loved one in dealing with the varied and difficult symptoms involved, as well as the coping strategies and treatments available. The next chapter will look in more detail at the practical ways you can help with everyday life.

CHAPTER 4

Practical Advice on How You Can Help with Everyday Life

CFS/ME has an impact on every area of a sufferer's life and this chapter aims to provide ideas for practical help that you can use to support your friend or relative with daily life. The subjects in this chapter will be most relevant for people who see their loved one regularly or daily, but even if you only see them occasionally the suggestions given will, it is hoped, ensure you can support them during the time you are with them, and understand their situation better.

As mentioned earlier in the book, it is important to remember that everyone is different and no two relationships work in the same way. While some of the advice given may be helpful to one person, if you or your loved one would not be comfortable with the suggestion made then it should be avoided. Pressurising someone or yourself to do something both or one of you are not comfortable with will not help anyone: it is important to do what feels right for you and your relationship. It is also important not to make assumptions about what your friend or family member needs. How they are and what you can do to help them will change over time, and if you keep asking them what is best for them as well as being honest about what you can offer, it will make life easier for both of you.

PERSONAL HYGIENE

Even the most basic everyday activities are affected by CFS/ME, and it is important to understand how the symptoms can compromise a person's ability to look after their appearance and get ready for the day. The physical effort involved in showering can require resting afterwards (even for people with mild CFS/ME), and some find that brushing their hair becomes impossible due to a lack of strength in their arms. The mental and physical effort required in washing clothes, ironing and then putting them away, and even deciding what to wear, makes these jobs sometimes impossible to do. Even making telephone calls to book dental or hairdressing appointments can be a challenge and lead to these self-care activities being avoided, which can further damage self-esteem.

How you can help

- Ask if they would like you to help with any of these things: brushing their hair, running them a bath, choosing outfits for them to wear over the next few days, making sure the washing and ironing is done, freshening the covers on their bed, putting fresh towels in the bathroom, ensuring there is a good stock of toilet paper.

- Help them with little things like making sure cosmetic bottles, shampoos and soaps are in easy-to-open containers. Making everything you can think of as easy as possible ensures that your friend or relative's energy is not being wasted on trying to open fiddly cosmetic bottles. Also keep an eye on when toiletries run out and make sure they are on a shopping list.

- Help them take care of themselves by making appointments on their behalf for the hairdresser or find a good one that does home visits if they would like this.

Sam, 35, has had CFS/ME moderately and severely at different stages, and explains:

> You feel dizzy and unsafe getting to the bathroom so you do not have a shower. You then have a quick wash at the sink. You get breakfast and lunch on autopilot while feeling in another place. Simple tasks become too much.

For severely affected sufferers, being able to wash, brush hair and teeth and even go to the toilet can become impossible to do without help, and this may result in needing full-time care, or even going into hospital or a care home. This is an extremely frightening and isolating experience and if your loved one is this ill it may be hard for you to understand, partly because they will find communicating this fear to you difficult. It will be very important to them to know that people are there for them.

Vanessa, 36, describes the intensive support she needed when she was severely ill:

> I would not have got through my ordeal without the support and love from my family and friends. It makes me tearful now as I think about the sacrifices they made for me. I couldn't be left alone and just them being there and their determination to help helped me to be strong and get through each hour, each day. My advice to relatives and friends is to appear strong even if underneath you are crumbling with the pressure, make a rota so you can have a break from caring, or you can make yourself ill too. A CFS patient is very hard to understand because there aren't really any ways to describe what you feel like.

FOOD AND NUTRITION

Food and nutrition are a vital part of everyone's health and well-being, and CFS/ME can have big practical implications as shopping, cooking and even eating can at times be very difficult or impossible. Any illness that involves fatigue can also benefit from some basic ideas about how to eat for maximising energy, which is also covered in this section.

Problems with eating

As with many health problems, there are issues to do with eating which are either directly caused by the condition or are a side-effect of the symptoms. Understanding that these are very real difficulties will help you to support your loved one to manage and eat as well as possible.

Digestive problems

Symptoms such as cramping stomach pain, wind, bloating, and alternating diarrhoea and constipation are often reported in people with CFS/ME, which are considered to be irritable bowel syndrome (IBS) and can make eating difficult, with symptoms flaring up after eating. Some people identify particular types of foods as causing them a problem, such as intolerance of dairy products, and the yeast infection *candida albicans*, or thrush, is also experienced by many sufferers, which has unpleasant symptoms. If they are having any of these problems your loved one may be following an exclusion diet of some type or on medication that has been advised as a way of managing and minimising these problems.

Difficulties chewing and swallowing

Some sufferers experience problems with their throats that can feel tight and restricted, making breathing and swallowing difficult. They may avoid certain foods or eating with other people to manage this.

Relying on 'junk' or low-nutrition foods

This is a common problem for busy people who don't have time to cook, or who are on a low income, but even more so with CFS/ME. This is because they may be physically unable to prepare complex meals. The cravings for high-energy foods that occur with extreme fatigue can make it difficult to eat healthily. Eating mainly processed high-fat and high-sugar foods can actually make the fatigue experienced in CFS/ME worse.

Having a poor appetite

Some people with CFS/ME lose a lot of weight as they feel so ill they are unable to eat. If this is the case supplements or medical help may be required to prevent malnutrition.

Preparing and making food at home

Choosing food, standing to prepare it, chopping the ingredients, opening jars and concentrating on cooking can all be problems to different degrees at various stages of the illness.

How you can help

- Help them choose the food for the next few meals, the ingredients required and if possible help them by preparing some of the ingredients in advance.

- Ready-chopped vegetables are quick, but lose some of their nutrients after preparation, and can be expensive. Frozen or tinned fruit and vegetables can be a useful quick, cheaper and nutritious alternative. Some of the time-saving chopping gadgets on the high street may reduce the effort required in making meals. Easy tin openers and a stool for sitting on while preparing and cooking the food are also very helpful.

- If you can help out with the actual cooking, for example making more than you need and freezing some for another day, then this would be hugely welcome, especially if your friend or family member lives alone.

- To ensure their overall diet is healthy and nutritious, sit down with your friend or relative and work out a weekly meal plan. This will not only help them when it comes to shopping, but it will also highlight when they might need help preparing food, when food could be made in double quantities (and so put in the freezer) and if there is anything lacking in their diet.

- Make sure they have healthy snacks to hand. Replace some of their high-sugar or high-fat snacks with healthier options, such as fruit, nuts or even a tub of frozen yoghurt!

Social eating

Eating out with friends and family can be an enjoyable way to spend time together, but when someone has CFS/ME some aspects of this become very problematic. Social eating can be noisy and exciting, making some people with CFS/ME very anxious about participating in these outings, even if they are being held at a friend's house. The combined extra stimulation, whether positive or negative, can over-stretch mental energy and increase adrenaline levels, making the symptoms of CFS/ME worse, either there and then, or the following day. Your loved one may not feel able to be honest about this, so anticipating and accepting that there may be some difficulties will be appreciated.

How you can help

- Appreciate that it is taking a great deal of energy for your friend or relative to participate and ensure they are happy and comfortable.

- Try to keep the number of people present relatively small so they are not overwhelmed.

- Try to keep it a bit quieter than usual. Understand that there will be so much going on (the food, the conversation), and try to ensure that the music is not too loud.

- Dim the lights so a calmer atmosphere is created.

- Subtly make sure your friend or relative knows they can leave whenever they wish, or even lie down in a quieter room in the house, and that you would not be offended.

Food and energy management

As you will know yourself, being very tired can lead to cravings for high-energy or sugary foods or highly caffeinated drinks such as coffee or cola. These are all commonly used methods for extending limited energy but because low energy is a constant problem in CFS/ME, reliance on these things can become habit and ultimately unhealthy. Caffeine and sugary foods and drinks can also increase dips in energy, so having an understanding of alternative ways of maximising and managing limited energy can really help someone with CFS/ME. Some specialists recommend eating foods that are absorbed slowly by the body to help stabilise energy, thus reducing the depth of energy slumps (common, for example, after eating a heavy lunch or highly processed meal). The Glycaemic Index (GI) (see Leeds *et al.* 2003) is a ranking of carbohydrates based on their effect on blood sugar levels and, broadly speaking, the closer foods are to their natural unprocessed state, the lower their glyceamic value is, which is better for sustained energy (with some exceptions). By using the GI system no foods are excluded from someone's diet, but instead you are developing an awareness of how different foods affect the body. If your family member or friend with CFS/ME is interested in incorporating the GI system into their diet, you may need to support them with the changes it will create in their shopping and cooking habits. It is not unknown for people with CFS/ME to make several dietary changes over a period of time to try and manage their symptoms.

CASE STUDY: JAMES

James, 35, explains how he did this when he first became moderately to severely ill with CFS/ME:

I did an anti-*candida* diet for a few months, to see whether there was lingering bacteria that might be perpetuating the fatigue, or posing a barrier to recovery. This meant I cut out, or drastically reduced, sugar and yeast. I also reduced other foodstuffs that might have either accelerated my collapse or mitigate against its recovery. Caffeine – which formerly sustained me through long workdays – was out, and herbal teas in. Fortunately, I lost my taste for alcohol, except for the odd glass of red wine.

It is important that loved ones respect and support any changes that someone chooses to make. In most cases the changes being made are the result of research they have carried out on the subject and the illness. However, if you have serious concerns about something that seems drastic, be careful about how you communicate this to them. Don't forget that they are probably desperate to feel better and that the illness affects the body in ways that you haven't experienced, so instead of criticising them try to understand the reasoning behind any changes that seem radical to you.

How you can help

- Support their decision to reduce certain foods and try not to eat too much of something they are not having in front of them.

- Help them research the glycaemic index diet and work out which foods are the most helpful for them.

- Help them to find new foods to replace the ones they have reduced. Better still, you could learn together about alternative health foods (such as tofu, quinoa, miso soup and soya) and have fun cooking a meal with the new foods.

Supplements

Sometimes extravagant claims are made for expensive nutritional supplements being helpful, and even righting imbalances in people with CFS/ME. There is no conclusive proof that any of these are effective treatments for the condition, and although some people feel that they have helped them, it is wise to be wary of anything promising amazing results unless this is backed up by research. Specialists working with CFS/ME recommend healthy eating, including plenty of fresh fruit and vegetables, as the best way to maximise nutrient intake and energy management.

Drinking

ALCOHOL

Many people with CFS/ME report becoming intolerant of alcohol; others find that because they have such difficulties already with sleep and fatigue, drinking alcohol affects them more than before they were ill. Alcohol interferes with deep sleep, which can already be in short supply, so your loved one may decide to reduce or stop drinking alcohol completely. Try to understand that this may be a big change to make; you could support them with this decision by reducing how much you drink around them and not pressurising them into drinking.

HYDRATION

Another important factor in energy management is drinking enough liquid to keep the brain and body well hydrated. Even mild dehydration can have an impact on the symptoms of CFS/ME, contributing to fatigue, concentration problems, headaches and dizziness. Dehydration has already started once a person becomes thirsty, and the colour of urine is the best way to identify whether you are drinking enough (ideally it should be a pale straw colour). Water or herbal teas are useful to help you drink enough liquid, but water in food also contributes to hydrating the body (for example, the water absorbed in rice during cooking). Alcohol, sugary and caffeinated drinks can contribute to symptoms and energy problems as they can affect blood sugar levels, over-stimulate the nervous system and encourage urine production rather than hydration, so are best drunk sparingly. If you see your loved one regularly you can help by encouraging them to find drinks they enjoy and reminding them to keep sipping regularly throughout the day. It is also important to be careful not to drink too much liquid, as this can be dangerous. A guide is between one and a half and two litres a day.

SHOPPING

The majority of modern shopping is done in big supermarkets or malls which are usually busy, noisy, vast places with lots of choice. When you are well these can be convenient, time-saving, even enjoyable experiences. But with CFS/ME completing a shopping trip can feel like trying to climb Mount Everest! In order to understand why shopping is so difficult for someone with CFS/ME, consider the following factors from the viewpoint of your family member or friend with the illness.

Factors to consider

Planning

Planning involves making lists, checking cupboards, remembering what you need, trying to work out how to go at less busy times. All these processes take energy and concentration, increasing fatigue and other symptoms before the shopping trip even starts.

Travelling to the shop

Whether driving or using public transport, travel is a major undertaking in CFS/ME and can use up a lot of your loved one's energy.

Walking round the shop

Walking when shopping is harder than walking at a regular pace because stopping and standing places greater demands on the heart as it pumps blood around the body. This can cause an increase in many of the symptoms such as leg aching, fatigue, feelings of weakness, palpitations and feeling faint, which altogether or even on their own can be very frightening and unpleasant.

Meeting people you know

Bumping into people you know in the shops can fill someone with CFS/ME with dread. Not only does it require more standing and increase the time taken to finish the shopping, it can also be hard concentrating on the conversation with so much going on around you as well as having to answer questions about how you are. In such a public and busy place, providing answers to such questions can be very draining as well as distressing to talk about.

Finding the items on your list

As you go round the shop, energy levels drop and the cognitive problems the illness causes can get in the way of the task. Difficulties processing information and focusing (brain fog) can make linking the items on the list and the items on the shelves very difficult, with the written words becoming meaningless. It can feel like the hardest thing you have ever had to do – to carry on when your body and mind are screaming for rest. This is also petrifying because it is natural to fear that this level of disability must be caused by a major brain disease or mental illness. Even when you know logically this is not the case the experience is so extreme that at times it is very difficult to be reassured when you are no longer able to find the biscuits in a supermarket.

Browsing

Similarly, browsing for gifts or other things you need to spend time choosing, such as clothes, brings the same problems. It hurts, increases fatigue and is very frustrating. This may also lead to increased anxiety because needing to buy a particular thing and finding it so hard to do so increases feelings of pressure, in turn increasing adrenaline levels and so symptoms.

Finishing the job

Many times you might find that it just isn't possible to finish the shopping, that you have to give up and go home. This will then cause other problems when you end up without the things you need as well as feeling frustrated and upset that you haven't been able to do something you had set out to do.

Standing in a queue to pay

By this point a combination of aching, malaise, confusion, pain, headache, dizziness and exhaustion can make standing in a queue to pay very difficult. Things such as checking you have been charged the right amount and packing the shopping safely can get lost in the desperation for it all to be over as soon as possible.

Carrying bags / unloading the trolley

Lifting and carrying are difficult for various reasons in CFS/ME – aching and de-conditioned muscles, as well as weakness and fatigue, all place extra demands on a person's energy stores. As this task comes at the end of the shop, you can appreciate it becomes even harder to do.

Travelling home again

The difficulties getting to the shop are magnified afterwards, and may make the sufferer feel at risk, as the ability to concentrate on crossing roads safely or drive is reduced. The trip may have exhausted and exceeded all energy reserves, leaving nothing left to get home again.

Unpacking when you get home

The relief of returning home again and the overwhelming need for rest can mean there is not enough energy to lift a kettle to make a drink, so unpacking the shopping may not get done for some time.

CASE STUDY: 'FRAN'

'Fran', 35, who had moderate CFS/ME, says:

> I often had the surreal and frightening experience of standing in an aisle of a familiar shop with a list in my hand and not being able to connect the words on the list with the item on the shelf right in front of me. Afterwards, sitting in a supermarket car park crying from the combination of exhaustion, frustration and pain was a frequent thing. The relief of being able to sit down at last combined with the fact that I would then have to rest for at least half an hour before I had the strength to drive the one mile home made me even more upset.

The symptoms experienced while shopping can continue for the rest of the day as well as interrupt that night's sleep with additional pain and extra adrenaline surging around the body. For the following few days, sufferers can experience an increase in symptoms as a result of one shopping trip. Professional athletes are sometimes advised by their trainers not to go shopping before a big event as it is considered to be such a drain on precious energy! This helps to explain why even when other demanding activities are possible for people with CFS/ME and they are improving overall, shopping can still be very difficult.

How you can help

- Help with the planning and making a list. Go through their cupboards with them as well as what they need for the week ahead and add it to a shopping list. Keeping a running list can also save time and energy.

- Go shopping with them, and if they get tired, make sure they rest while you finish the shop. Making sure the supermarket or town centre you are going to has a café can be very important as it means there is always somewhere where your friend can go if they get too tired while you finish the shopping.

- Help them carry the bags and unpack the shopping afterwards.

- Encourage them to consider internet shopping, even for groceries, which can be done when they are up to it (or by someone else) and delivered at a time when you or another friend or family member will be around to help them unpack.

- When you pop to the shops, call them and ask if there is anything they need as you are going anyway. While it wouldn't be much extra trouble for you, it could be a lifeline to them. Carol, 64, has had CFS/ME for 29 years and wishes for 'shopping to be done for me (without me having to think what to buy!)'.

MOBILITY AND TRAVEL

When you have CFS/ME, getting around can become very complicated. However, you can support your loved one by helping them find new ways of doing things. This can involve a big change in your role when you are with them as they concentrate on managing the small details of being out and about. People who get disabled persons benefits in the UK are also entitled to passes to use public transport for free. Schemes vary in other countries; please see the disability and benefits organisations listed in the Resources section for information.

Driving

Some people with mild or moderate CFS/ME find that driving becomes a major difficulty; for people with severe CFS/ME it is impossible. Driving requires high levels of concentration and split-second decision making with frequent surges of adrenaline while in a static position. As you have probably come to realise from reading this book, the physical and cognitive symptoms of CFS/ME may make driving very difficult, increasing tension, muscle aches, headaches and levels of fatigue. This may mean your loved one has to give up driving altogether.

How you can help

- If you are able to give lifts, do so.

- Try to park closer to the place you are going or drop them off near somewhere to sit while you park the car.

- Find alternative modes of transport for them.

- Draw up a rota with other family members or friends to help with transport.

- If they decide to continue driving, share the driving as much as possible.

Things that seem small to you can greatly enhance the quality of life of someone with a chronic illness. So if you are very busy and don't see what you can do to help, ask if there is anything small you can do to help them. Berni says 'getting a lift to somewhere lovely has been brilliant – for example, to my local park as I can't walk there anymore, but still want to be outside and see nature and hopefully have a short stroll'.

Parking

Parking can be difficult if you have CFS/ME because after driving for even a short time, levels of fatigue and pain can increase and there may be little energy left to park. In the UK, the Blue Badge scheme is available for people with mobility problems who have difficulty walking and using public transport, enabling them to have access to parking in limited places or close to services (see Resources section for details of this, and for similar schemes in other countries contact your local charity as listed or your local council). However, once a badge is obtained, a person with CFS/ME may have problems using it. They may feel embarrassed; or that it means they are accepting their limitations and have given up on returning to full health; or uncomfortable at the ignorance of others who see someone with CFS/ME getting out of their car and walking and assume that they don't have a disability.

How you can help

- Help them to see that these schemes are there for people in their situation to help make life easier, and that their quality of life is a priority.

- Be aware of any reservations they may have and reassure your loved one of their right to the available travel schemes in order to help them get around.

- Go with them to practice using these parking spaces until they feel more comfortable.

Buses

Travelling on buses has many hidden difficulties for someone with CFS/ME, starting before they even get on the bus. It may become their main way of getting around as reduced income and difficulties driving make other methods less accessible.

Waiting for the bus

You may not have noticed that only some bus stops have seats, and when they do they are often busy. Knowing that after a short period of time your legs will begin to ache and the effort of standing will begin to make you feel breathless can increase anxiety even before it has an impact on symptoms. Also, if the bus is for a return journey and fatigue levels are already high, having to stand for a return bus can be the final straw and tip energy levels into deficit. Planning journeys on public transport is hard when some routes are not reliable.

Getting a seat

Busy buses present a challenge for most people with CFS/ME. Their difficulties are hidden to others as they may look 'well', so people are unlikely to offer to give up a seat for them. Asking if you can have someone else's seat is very difficult as it feels as though an explanation is required and this may be an emotional thing to have to do. It is difficult enough to explain the illness to a friend, let alone a stranger. A walking stick can be a useful symbol of disability in public situations, can be useful to lean on and may encourage other people to give up their seat.

How you can help

- Find up-to-date information on useful bus routes and ensure your friend or family member has the correct times and fare information.

- If you are with them, ask someone if your friend or family member can have a seat as they are not well.

Taxis

Travelling by taxi can be a helpful way to get around as it avoids the difficulties of driving, parking and timing public transport. But for most people with CFS/ME the cost will mean they can only be an occasional luxury.

How you can help

- Make sure your friend or family member has the number of a few taxi companies and spare cash on them at all times. They can be helpful when they can no longer deal with a return journey home on public transport, reducing the impact on their symptoms.

- Ensure your friend or family member always has a mobile phone on them (with a charged battery!) as well as a list of people they can contact in an emergency at different times of the day. Having this list on them can make them feel more confident in going out as there is always someone that can come and help them should they get into difficulties.

Travelling long distances

Sitting still for long periods of time, whether in a car, train or bus, can be very difficult as the stiffness of muscles and pain can increase. Travel can also increase anxiety when delays, changes and noise levels are out of our control and a sufferer can feel their symptoms getting worse.

How you can help

- Help your loved one to assess all aspects of any travel plans to try and work out the least difficult, quickest or quietest route.

Trains and planes

Train and aeroplane travel have many hidden difficulties for someone with CFS/ME. For the majority that do not use a wheelchair, standing in long queues at ticket desks and check-in can be very tiring and make them feel ill before the trip has even begun. There are never enough seats for all passengers when waiting to board a plane. Even for people who are using a wheelchair, the bright lights, noise and busyness of a terminal or station can easily be too much.

Queuing is very difficult for people with CFS/ME because it involves muscle strength in their legs and the heart has to work harder when standing still, increasing feelings of dizziness and fatigue. However, there are things that can be done to reduce the impact of these things.

Assisted travel schemes

Most travel companies have a policy to assist disabled travellers when using their services. Even mildly affected people who don't consider themselves disabled but have problems with queuing, standing and waiting for long periods can benefit from assistance. Help and adaptations can be made to the checking in process, bypassing queues, having somewhere to sit and wait, and assistance getting on and off the mode of transport, transfers and help carrying baggage. All of this can be arranged ahead of time.

How you can help

- If your friend or family member is happy for you to do this, offer to explain to staff at airports and railway stations what their needs and problems are. Sometimes the main barrier to getting help is the embarrassment and distress felt as well as the difficulty explaining a complex situation to a stranger. Any support or assistance you can offer regarding this would be hugely appreciated by your friend or relative.

- Better still, contact the airline or rail company in advance to discuss your loved one's needs and arrange what they can offer.

Mobility aids

Walking, standing and queuing are problems for all CFS/ ME sufferers, and mobility aids can be a great help when pacing energy and preventing severe setbacks. Wheelchairs are useful even when a person can walk short distances, by conserving energy, reducing pain and minimising the risk of symptoms as an after-effect of going out.

However, the use of mobility aids like walking sticks and wheelchairs represents the crossing of a line that is very emotive. Going from invisible to visible disability means a change in how others see you, and can also mean a shift in how a person sees themselves. They may feel that it means the illness has beaten them, contributing to low mood and possibly depression.

CASE STUDY: 'MELANIE'

'Melanie', 31, who has moderate CFS/ME, says:

> I used a chair stick when I knew that I would not be able to stay at the event I was going to without it, for example, going to watch a friend run a five-kilometre race on a wet day, or a day in a city I hadn't been to before and didn't know where I would be able to sit and rest. Every time I stood at the front door I was torn between leaving it behind and appearing 'normal' and taking it and having to deal with the fact that it made me stand out from the crowd. If I was with friends I was sometimes pleased to have physical evidence that I was seriously ill, it helped them to understand that it hurt me to stand up. I used humour to cope with these different feelings, referring to it as my 'cripple chair', which shows how it made me feel. There were many more times when I didn't take it that I needed it, and ended up having to sit on the floor of shops, at the sides of roads because I was in too much pain and too breathless to continue. But at the time I would rather do that than take my chair stick with me because it upset me too much.

The negative ways people can react to and treat wheelchair users is well known: ignoring, patronising and avoiding them, adding to the isolation and emotional struggle that coping with any illness already brings. In moderate CFS/ME the use of a wheelchair or scooter needs to be finely balanced, as for a sufferer to use it all the time and stop walking completely will contribute to further deterioration of the condition through lack of use of the muscles. In addition to this, having a wheelchair that is sometimes used and walking the rest of the time can be difficult as a sufferer will be aware how other people might respond to someone who is using a chair and yet can also be seen to walk.

CASE STUDY: SAM

'Sam', 35, expresses her struggle with mobility:

> I suffered repeatedly when doing what looks like to others a low-key outing; this ultimately led to wheelchair/scooter use for certain things. This came as a shock to my husband because he did not believe it was necessary for a while. I have to say that using a wheelchair or scooter to save energy prevents the setbacks. I do shorter things on foot and often use the walking-stick-seat for a queue. I use my walking-stick-seat for familiar ground when I know the timescale involved.

People with the most severe levels of CFS/ME, when they are well enough to go out, are unable to leave the house without the assistance of a wheelchair or mobility scooter. For people who are less severely affected the issue of help while getting around is a complex one, as while they may have a very restricted ability to walk, they can do so, even though this will often mean pain and huge effort. Despite this, for many people with the illness, the fact that they are able to walk can mean that relatives, their doctor, carers and friends may not consider all the options for making their life easier.

How you can help

- Talk through with them any reasons for avoiding using the mobility aids that may help them.

- Support them to use their legal rights to assistance by encouraging them to accept what they are entitled to.

- Advocate on their behalf if they want you to.

- Help them to get more information on the options and choices available – see Resources section for organisations specialising in mobility aids.

- Be aware of any uncomfortable feelings you may have about them using a chair or other aids that draws attention to their illness. This can be a difficult change for you too and may lead to feelings of embarrassment, self-consciousness and anger. If you feel this way make sure you talk it through with your friend or another person you are close to.

- Try to see that mobility aids are a positive tool, increasing a person's abilities and enjoyment by reducing symptoms.

DOMESTIC TASKS, DIY AND GARDENING

Even apparently simple household tasks such as washing up, vacuuming, ironing and cleaning can be very difficult for someone with CFS/ME as, like shopping, they place multiple demands on the body's stamina, involving standing and physical exertion, resulting in increased pain and malaise. Also, as these tasks are often perceived as 'easy to do' activities, people with CFS/ME are likely to place demands on themselves to do them even though they create so much discomfort and suffering.

'Sam', 35, explains that when her illness has been milder and she has been able to work, other things have still been a struggle:

Socialising can still be low key, as can be the amount of housework you can be well enough for. Things still had the potential to build up. At that point I judged my health on if the bathroom was cleaned that week and the laundry was done.

How you can help

- It is very important that you understand which domestic chores your loved one has difficulties with; what one person with CFS/ME struggles with may not be the same as another. This may not always seem logical – the random and changeable nature of symptoms often doesn't make sense to a sufferer either.

- Try not to assume that because they are doing something it is not causing them any problems.

- If you are avoiding asking them about the domestic chores be honest with yourself: are you worried you might have to take on some of their responsibilities and are unsure how you will cope? If this is the case, discuss the matter with other friends or family members to see if other people can help as well. If this isn't possible, organise a schedule that fits in with your available time for when chores get done.

- If your friend or family member wishes to keep on doing domestic chores despite the problems it may bring, respect their decision as it is a way of them trying to stay independent. However, it is important they pace themselves. Discuss with them ways they can break tasks into smaller activities and reduce the number of activities in one day. This may take a lot of patience and understanding from you but it is important that they are supported to have some independence and gain a sense of achievement. Working with them to find new ways of dividing up tasks that suits you both is important to try and avoid resentment building up.

'Fran', 35, who has moderate CFS/ME, explains:

> I did the washing up in three sections if I was having a 'bad day', resting for a few minutes between each part and this stopped me getting utterly exhausted and reduced the pain in my legs and arms. It was hard to accept that I should do this to start with, but I felt *less* useless when I had finished.

Be aware that with you offering to do some or many of their domestic chores, your friend or relative with CFS/ME may start to feel frustrated and embarrassed. It is a delicate balancing act of helping but not taking over! The best way to ensure no feelings of failure or resentment build up is to talk openly with your friend or relative, asking what they would like to do rather than taking over and doing everything. It can be useful to have a standing arrangement so that they don't have to keep asking for help and you both know where you stand.

MONEY, EMPLOYMENT AND WORK

It is important to realise that for many people who become seriously ill their financial situation changes dramatically and in many cases they have to rely on benefits. This will, of course, change their standard of living, and have big implications for their future security. This can lead to anger, frustration, embarrassment and depression. Money problems may well affect what they are able to do socially, as they have to become more careful. It can also change the balance of your relationship with them as their lifestyle changes and they are forced to alter their perspective on what is important in life.

Sick pay

If your friend or family member is off sick from work, they may be entitled to sick pay. This will be related to their length of service and is often restricted to a set period of time, reducing after a few months and eventually stopping completely. This can add to a person's stress levels and put pressure on them to try to return to previous levels of activity. They may worry that they will have to retire on medical grounds if they are unable to return to work within the period expected by their employer and may need support with finding out about policies and procedures. Check with the employer for details.

Insurance

Payment protection insurance (PPI), income protection, mortgage and credit card insurance are all commonly held policies that can include cover for periods of chronic illness. Becoming seriously ill and struggling to function can sometimes mean that people forget insurance policies that they have or don't realise that they cover their current circumstances. It is worth checking if your loved one has any of these as they can make the difference between high levels of anxiety and taking the pressure off, even temporarily.

State benefits

There are specific financial schemes in the UK that some people with CFS/ME are entitled to such as Disability Living Allowance and Employment and Support Allowance. Some apply even when a person already has other money coming in. Benefits can be difficult for someone with CFS/ ME to acquire as the criteria can be very specific, and the claim forms are complicated and time consuming, making them a challenge for someone with concentration problems and fatigue. Sometimes an initial claim is turned down due to errors in the application or reasons that are unclear. It is worth getting advice and applying again – people with CFS/ ME can find that they are awarded on the second or even third attempt. It can be useful to get help with working out entitlement and how to apply, and as benefits systems vary between countries, see the Resources section for government helplines and independent organisations offering advice specific to your country.

How you can help

- Be sensitive to the fact that money will probably be an issue for your loved one when you are planning social occasions, presents, holidays, etc. You could ask them what they want to do instead of assuming things will be the same as ever.

- If you feel confident to do this you could offer to help to find out what they are entitled to by phoning helplines or going with them to get advice.

- Benefits change frequently so it is important you keep checking the guidelines and procedures on government websites to ensure your friend or relative is claiming what they are entitled to.

- The benefits system can seem uncaring and judgemental when you are ill so it is important to have supportive people to help you negotiate it. Seeking help from loved ones, a Disability Rights Advisor via an employer, a disability charity as listed in the

Resources section, or an independent benefits advice charity can make the process a lot less upsetting.

- You could help them to complete claim forms by reading the small print for them and breaking the process down into smaller sections to work on over a few sessions; this will help them to concentrate and reduce the impact on symptoms.

- Help them to focus on answering each question with brief and relevant information only. However tempting it is to make other points these will not be taken into account and may go against them. There is often an additional information section at the end for the other things they wish to say.

- If your loved one has difficulty writing due to pain or concentration problems you can complete the form on their behalf.

- Supporting them to have a good relationship with one doctor, if at all possible, can be important when medical reports for benefits and other help are required. The better the GP knows them, the more accurate and detailed the information they can provide in support of any claims.

- If they have not been awarded a benefit they seemed to be entitled to, understand that the frustration, stress and upset of this and going through appeals procedures and medical assessments is very real, and can also have a negative impact on their physical symptoms. This can mirror their experience of people not believing that they are ill and is very distressing.

- Know that it is difficult to be assertive and stand up for your rights when you have CFS/ME as it saps your energy and concentration, making tasks that you might take for granted seem impossible, and help valuable.

- You could help them by offering to make any difficult phone calls on their behalf to explain the situation while they are with you, and pass the phone over to them if needed. This may help reduce their stress levels and help them concentrate for long enough.

- If they are employed, find out if their employer has a Disability Rights Advisor; large organisations have Equality and Diversity and Occupational Health departments that can be an invaluable source of support on benefits, rights and return to work issues.

Work

Having a sense of purpose in life is often tied up in a working role, whether paid, voluntary, learning, caring or parenting, and CFS/ME threatens this important aspect of life at every level. In the majority of CFS/ME cases (77%) the sufferer has to stop organised work or studying either because they are physically unable to continue, or because adaptations that could be carried out are not made by employers (Action for ME 2006). Having CFS/ME will mean short, medium and long-term changes to working life, and if these can be tackled one step at a time without assuming that the person's work life is over completely, this will benefit everyone. In the UK, The Disability Discrimination Act (1995/2005) supports the right of a worker with CFS/ME to have 'reasonable adjustments' made to their role in order to be able to sustain it. Other legislation supports the rights of employees with disabling conditions in other counties; contact your local disability charity for information.

The threat of losing your job or this actually happening has huge implications for self-esteem, sense of future security and overall coping with having CFS/ME. Anything employers, managers and colleagues can do to support someone will benefit the sufferer immensely. It is recognised by some experts that having a positive focus and support for coping from your workplace can have a big influence on whether someone recovers from CFS/ME. Be careful not to make assumptions about your friend and family member working, because, as the following example shows, being able to work does not necessarily mean everything is back to how it was.

'Sam', 35, has had CFS/ME fluctuating between severe and moderate levels:

> My condition has taken different forms. In earlier times I did return to work part time. That was until a relapse. However that also impacted upon people's perceptions of how I could manage in between times. If you are (so called) lucky enough to be well enough to work part time, then people can need a lot of persuasion to understand that it takes a lot of energy and there is little left. People assume that if you are well enough to work, then you are well enough to get back to everything else, as though there is little wrong with you.

People who have mild CFS/ME, or are in the early stages of the illness, usually manage to keep working or studying despite very low levels of energy and stamina, concentration problems, aches and generally feeling rough. This has a big impact on their home life and leisure time, which often becomes the time when they have to conserve their energy, shrinking domestic and leisure activities and changing their family relationships.

People with moderate CFS/ME may well have long periods of time off sick from work or find that they can no longer sustain their role in its current form. It may be possible for changes to be made to working hours, patterns, roles and responsibilities that mean they can stay in employment.

Those who experience severe CFS/ME may have a long time off sick from their work or may be retired on medical grounds, which is often not what they want to happen. However, some do return to working when they are improved, which may mean they still have the condition but in a less disabling form. Supporting someone who is in this position effectively is key to them sustaining employment, as their ability to work may depend on finding new ways of doing so and they may develop home working, freelance, or self-employed work in order to have the control they need to stay well and prevent relapse. Managers, Human Resources, Occupational Health Services and college course leaders may find people with CFS/ME difficult to manage, especially if they have no experience of dealing with the illness among their workforce. However, doing nothing is likely to make the situation worse, and because CFS/ME is legally recognised in the UK as a disability they have an obligation to consider making changes. Legislation in other countries provides a similar obligation; contact your local disability charity for information.

How you can help

- Discuss with your friend, relative or colleague what they would like to happen. They are likely to have many ideas about how they can continue to work while looking after themselves. It is important that they are clear about their needs and priorities so they can be fully involved in any decision making.

- Help them to consider a wide variety of possibilities for their work/life balance as what they need to manage life with CFS/ME will be very different from how things were before they became ill.

- Help them to plan discussion points for a meeting with their employer or help them to write a letter explaining to their manager, HR department or tutor about the illness, outlining a range of options that could be made to help them continue working.

- Possible options to consider include: flexible working hours (as long as the job is done by the end of the working week or day, the actual start and finish times are flexible to accommodate how the person is feeling); working from home to reduce the energy drain of travel; changing a role to job share or a part-time post; increasing the number of breaks; temporary reduced hours; regular reviews of both the employer and person with CFS/ME's needs, ensuring everyone is happy with the situation.

- See pp.79–83 for more on your relationship with a colleague who has CFS/ME.

CARING RESPONSIBILITIES

If your friend or relative with CFS/ME looks after other members of the family, it is important that everyone assesses whether this is still possible.

How you can help

- The first thing to do is to discuss with your loved one how they feel about their caring responsibilities and whether they would like help or changes to be made. It might be that they would like to continue with the caring role but would like help with other aspects of their life (shopping, domestic chores, etc.).

- In the UK, anyone who has a caring role is entitled to a Carer's Assessment, a detailed assessment of their needs, which is available from social services and can help you to find support options. For other countries, carers' charities can advise on rights and the support available in your area; see the Resources section for contact details.

- If they would like help with their caring activities, discuss the matter with other relatives and friends to see what can be done.

- There are a range of charities and support groups for carers that can help both you as the carer of someone with CFS/ME, and your loved one who has CFS/ME, if they in turn are a carer for someone else. See the Resources section for organisations and contact them to see what help and support they can offer.

CASE STUDY: JAY

Jay had severe CFS/ME and says:

> I never got any help from family or friends, they all just ran! What I would have liked to have happened was my daughter could have delegated the problem to get me carers, but I didn't know about such things. She was in sixth form boarding due to my illness and I was a single parent. I thought if I told social services I was bedridden my daughter and dog would be taken off me. If you haven't come in contact with social workers before you are simply afraid. If only I had known about care assessments and that not all social workers do is take your children off you.

SOCIALISING AND COMMUNICATION

When a loved one becomes ill with CFS/ME, it is useful to think about how you have kept in touch and socialised with them in the past, and consider whether this is still the best way to keep your relationship going. This will especially be the case if they have usually been the one who rings, suggests meeting up or visits you, as it is unlikely that they will be able to continue to do these things in the same way. They will appreciate an honest conversation from you about how best to stay in touch as this will show that you care and understand that their illness is serious. When friends or family members say nothing and stay away it is easy for the sufferer to feel that they don't care and this can lead to relationships breaking down.

Amala says:

> Social isolation is a big challenge. Friends and family could really help fight it by connecting once a week or so via a phone, email, Instant Messaging or texting. When I am unable to attend parties or events because of energy limitations, it really helps me feel connected when friends and family send 'live' pictures from their phones.

Mild CFS/ME

People with mild CFS/ME are usually able to socialise but may find intense conversation more tiring than they used to. Energy levels are much lower than average and although your loved one may be able to work, they will find it hard to do things you take for granted, such as going to parties. Concentration is harder to maintain and socialising – even though enjoyable – can increase other symptoms.

How you can help

- Ask if they would like to change the way you spend time together to make it easier for them. This could mean doing something different or for a shorter time. For example: if they have always made food for you when you go to their home, it will be helpful now for you to ask if they want to do anything differently as the complexity and effort that goes into entertaining will seriously deplete their energy and may affect them for days after you have gone.

- Find new ways of keeping in touch. Long telephone conversations are often difficult for people with CFS/ME so you could use email instead as this would let them reply when they are feeling up to it, or keep your chats shorter.

- Try to find new activities that they are able to manage. For example, if you are eating out, plan where you are going and how to get there in advance because walking around for long periods looking for a restaurant will cause discomfort.

Moderate CFS/ME

For people with moderate CFS/ME, socialising will be more difficult but as they may no longer be working they may be feeling isolated, which makes any contact with friends and family even more important.

How you can help

- You may find that your friend or relative finds it harder to keep in touch with you so why not take more responsibility for this, asking them what they need from you to keep the relationship going.

- Discuss with them what they feel like doing and try not to push them into doing something you would like to do.

- When you are together at a social event, try to make it easier for them to enjoy themselves by helping them to take rests from the 'action' and be prepared for them to need to leave early as this will reduce the amount they suffer the following day.

- Text or email before you ring to check that they are feeling up to chatting on the phone, or to arrange a suitable time.

Severe CFS/ME

For severely affected people CFS/ME will have completely changed their life and the loss of contact with others is one of its cruellest effects. At its worst, severe CFS/ME can mean that your friend is too ill to speak, see people or even read. The condition is very difficult for others to understand and sometimes it is easier to avoid someone than try to talk to them about it. If your relationship is important to you please try to find a way to keep in contact, they will be grateful! Sometimes keeping in touch via their main carer will be helpful.

Jane, 33, who has severe CFS/ME, says:

> During the worst stages of my illness I was too exhausted to email, speak on the phone or have visitors, so good communication between my main carer and friends/family was key in order for them to gain some understanding of what I was going through.

How you can help

- If you don't see your friend as much as you used to, let them know you care in the old-fashioned way: send them a card or letter of support and state your wish to stay in touch, but on their terms. If you don't get a quick response, try not to take it personally; it may well be that they would love to reply but are too ill to do so. This often changes over time so don't give up.

- Seeing a friend so ill and finding that they are unable to spend time with you is difficult. Work with them to work out ways of staying in touch they can manage, maybe visiting them, and staying for a shorter period of time.

- You may find yourself doing a lot for your loved one as they are struggling to manage. Make sure that they are comfortable with how you are spending time with them by asking them what they want from you. Do not assume that they are happy with your ideas as it may be difficult for them to question things when they are just grateful you are around. Maintaining a sense of control and independence is vital in CFS/ME as so much is lost through the illness and this can contribute to depression. You can help them by asking them what they need often as it will change over time.

James, 35, explains how difficult it can be for someone with moderate to severe CFS/ME to have a telephone conversation:

> If you are now living a rather isolated existence, you crave such human contact. But you're probably not up to a standard 20-minute conversation (particularly with five friends

per week), and both sufferer and friend need to understand this. If you're lucky enough to have someone screening calls for you (partner, parent), they can help you manage the unexpected incursion on your energy budget. If not, you need to be tough with yourself, and keep the chat duration within healthy limits.

Visiting

When going to visit your friend or family member, whether a regular thing or just once a year, everyone will benefit from thinking differently about things you probably took for granted in the past. For example: *when* you go, *how long* you stay, *how many people* come with you and *what* you talk about. It is hard to understand that sitting and talking can make someone feel more ill, but CFS/ME is a complex condition that can be affected by excitement and concentration as well as negative stress. It may affect them five minutes later or the next day, depending on their level of illness and whether they are having a good or a bad day, so the best thing to do is take your lead from them.

People with mild CFS/ME often seem no different, and it may only be those closest to them who can tell when they are struggling. This means that it is very important that you don't assume that they can do things the same as ever. For moderately affected people, your loved one may seem 'normal', but it is important that you try to understand that their stamina and energy for simple activities will be much less than before they were ill. Severe CFS/ME can mean the sufferer is too ill to sit up and speak. If they try to do activities that they have little energy for, it can result in a further deterioration in their condition meaning they suffer even more.

How you can help

- Ask them when you are arranging to meet how long they want to spend with you.

- Check that they are OK for you to stay every so often when you are there. It is hard to ask people to leave when you have had enough!

- Ask them well in advance what they would like to do and offer alternatives to your usual plans. For example, if they usually make all the food, ask if you can bring part or all of a meal and help to clean up afterwards.

- Take your cue from them and accept it if you are told that they are not up to seeing you. Remember it probably isn't anything personal, it is the illness!

When you are going to see your friend and family member in their home there are things to consider that apply across the spectrum of the illness. Jane, 33, who has been severely affected and is now improving, summarises them in these points (my additions in brackets):

- Arrange a day and time to visit. In the past, friends just showed up and most times I was resting or not well enough to see them. A text or phone call to arrange a suitable time is preferable. (Mornings can be the worst time of day for some sufferers as they struggle to get going, for others, evenings are the time their energy levels are at their lowest.)

- Don't be offended if your friend has to cancel. They will be far more disappointed than you, as you may be their only visitor that month! I usually arrange a visit in advance but on the understanding that I'll text on the day if I'm not well enough. (This is necessary as the symptoms can be very unpredictable day to day.)

- Try to be punctual. I once waited an exhausting two hours for a friend to show and when he did I was too ill to see him. I have to plan my regular rest periods around any visitors and if they don't show on time, my energy is depleting. Again, if you understand the illness a little you'll appreciate this.

- Try to keep visiting times short and stick to an agreed time. Time really does fly by, especially when you first start having visitors again, so much to catch up on! But it's better to see someone for a short time and perhaps often, than for exhausting hours and relapsing for weeks after.

Other factors to consider when visiting/socialising with people with moderate to severe CFS/ME

- Noise levels – music, children, loud voices, TV on in the background. People with moderate and severe levels of CFS/ME can find noise unbearable. It causes confusion and increases their fatigue so bear this in mind when you see them. Carol, 64, says that to help her cope with severe CFS/ME she would appreciate 'lowered voices, slower speech, gentle, quiet movements'.

- Concentration/memory problems – your loved one may find focusing on the conversation difficult and may struggle to recall words that they want to say, which they may find embarrassing. These can all be symptoms of the condition and your understanding and patience will be appreciated.

- Excitement and stimulating conversation can increase the levels of adrenaline in the system and contribute to exhaustion. They may need rest breaks even from having an enjoyable time.

- Perfume/aftershave/household deodorisers, etc. Some sufferers report adverse reactions to chemicals and strong smells, so consider not using your usual products when you see them if this applies to your loved one.

- Viral infections/colds – if you are ill or run down yourself, it is worth asking them if it is still OK to visit, as many people with CFS/ME report picking up infections easily, making their coping even harder.

What to talk about

Talking about your life and things your friend or relative with CFS/ME can't currently take part in (whether it be socially related, work related or plans for the future) may be difficult, so try to be sensitive to their situation when you are talking. If you are not sure how they are and what they can and can't do, don't assume, ask them! Generally they will want you to be yourself and not overly focus on their illness, but not ignore it either. It is about balance.

What to take

If you want to take a gift and are not sure what is suitable, ask their main carer or another friend or relative that sees them more regularly before you go. Traditional visiting gifts such as wine and chocolate may not be appreciated if your loved one has become intolerant of alcohol as many sufferers report, or are having problems with their weight. Consider fruit or other special food that they may be unable to shop for easily, or ask them if there is anything they need before you go. Or you could take something for them to do: a magazine or craft product.

Communication

As mentioned, people who have severe CFS/ME can be unable to read or write due to the overwhelming nature of their symptoms. Concentration and memory is compromised even in mild and moderate cases, making communication harder to take part in. Alongside the emotional impact on everyone, this makes your role in keeping good communication going even more important.

Being a good listener

Listening well is a skill. When we are having a conversation, we are often preparing what we are going to say next, or planning what we are doing later at the same time, which can mean that we don't listen fully. Really listening to someone in distress can be difficult and you may find yourself preoccupied with trying to think of ways to make them feel better, which may end up getting in the way of you actually hearing them. Consider these ideas:

- *Use open questions* to get enough information for you to understand them and also to encourage them to talk about difficult subjects. Asking someone '*how* they feel' or '*what* they want' rather than a closed question that only has a 'yes' or 'no' answer, opens up a discussion and allows your friend or relative to contribute as much or as little as they wish. It will also help you avoid assuming what they are experiencing is the same as last time you saw them, or how you think you would feel in their place. This is especially important in CFS/ME as the condition can be very changeable over time and even from one hour to the next.

- *Check that you have understood* by trying to communicate that you have heard how things are for them by summarising what they have said. This can be very useful if you are not sure that you have understood as it allows space for more information to be given. For example 'So, you are saying that…?' or 'Do you mean…?'

- *Be honest* if you are struggling to understand their situation or are feeling unsure about what you can do to help. Say so and you might be able to work it out together.

- *Don't doubt them* or question their symptoms. They may have faced a lot of disbelief already from doctors and other friends or relatives, so try not to question their integrity.

- *Acknowledge their distress and difficulties.* It can be tempting to just focus on the positives and trying to help them, but be careful that you don't seem to be minimising their problems by avoiding talking about them. This can hurt and leave someone with CFS/ME feeling misunderstood.

CONCLUSION

In this chapter we have looked at many areas of daily life, from personal hygiene to shopping, from food to employment, from domestic chores to mobility and the different problems that living with CFS/ME can bring. I hope I have also provided you with a wide range of suggestions to consider on how you can help and support your friend or relative with CFS/ME. The most important issue that comes up again and again is communication with your loved one: talk to them openly, find out their needs and where they would like help as well as respecting their sense of independence and personal achievement by allowing them to carry out some tasks themselves (if possible). Be sure to make sure you are taking care of your own needs too. It is all about balance and good communication and listening will help you and your loved one achieve this.

CHAPTER 5

The Top Ten Tips on How You Can Help

Finally, in the last chapter of the book, I want to bring together the most important ideas and information that are central to coping with having a loved one with CFS/ME. Included are the most frequent words of advice from loved ones of people with CFS/ME, who have helped sufferers adjust, to understand and even recover in some cases from this illness. They were asked 'What advice would you give to someone with a loved one with CFS/ME?' and their answers are echoed in the contributions from people with the illness.

If you don't have the time to read the whole book or want a final checklist of the key points in supporting your friend or relative, and looking after yourself while you do, then this chapter is for you.

1. LISTEN

- It is vital that you try to understand the *individual* experience of your loved one's illness and avoid making assumptions about CFS/ME and how it affects their life.

- Keep asking and keep listening because symptoms, energy levels and mobility problems are changeable at different times.

- Try to really understand how they feel, emotionally as well as physically, and your relationship with them will be easier to maintain.

'Millie', 35, friend of a moderately affected sufferer says:

> I hope that I have been understanding. This can be hard when there are no very obvious physical symptoms.

Millie overcame this by trying to imagine what it was like for her friend to live with CFS/ME and understand how it affected her everyday life, helping her to reduce the frustration she felt when they had to do things together more slowly than they used to.

2. ACCEPT

- Accept that they are seriously ill with a disabling and very distressing physical illness that affects every area of their life.

- Understanding that the implications of CFS/ME are far reaching, and accepting that it affects every tiny decision and action, will help you relate to the person in a more helpful way.

- Accept that they know best about how they feel because CFS/ME is very hard to describe to other people.

- If you can, accept and allow that they will be feeling some strong emotions and that these are a natural reaction to being physically ill.

- Accept that things have to change. Respecting whatever your friend tells you about how the condition affects them and their limitations, instead of trying to encourage them to carry on as normal, will help you to support them and adjust to the changes it brings. If you fight it too this will add to their difficulties.

3. LEARN

- Educating yourself about CFS/ME will give you a greater understanding of what they are facing. This may also be helpful for your friend or relative, as sometimes people get a diagnosis but no information about symptoms or how to cope.

- Try not to judge your loved one based on assumptions or small amounts of information you have heard about other people with CFS/ME. It is a very complex and variable condition.

- Subscribing to a CFS/ME-related newsletter, 'e-zine' or magazine, or finding a support group, may help those closest to a sufferer. See the Resources section for ideas.

Sairah, 35, friend of a moderately affected sufferer says:

> Encourage them to gain as much information as possible, and to learn to gauge and accept their limitations – and be aware that these will vary.

4. EXPECT CHANGE

- CFS/ME affects every area of a sufferer's life, and it will affect your relationship with them, too. Finding ways to adapt to the differences in how they can socialise and stay in touch can mean your relationship changes a lot, which can have both negative and positive effects.

- Flexibility is crucial. Going at their pace when you are with them might mean doing something in a very different way, maybe walking at a third of your usual speed, or waiting until they feel well enough to meet up instead of expecting to see them whenever you want to.

- Seeing things differently from the start will help you with this.

5. LOOK AFTER YOURSELF

- Watching someone you care about be seriously ill can be stressful, so it is important that you make sure you have support and information to help you cope.

- Ensure you have time for yourself to relax, eat and sleep well, and have regular breaks.

- Be kind to yourself and acknowledge that your loved one's illness affects you too.

May, 31, friend of a woman with moderate CFS/ME advises:

> Emotional support and an outlet for sufferers' frustrations with themselves and with their bodies is so important. If you can provide this – do. But look after yourself in the process and

make sure you have your own outlets, preferably to someone separate from the sufferer, who may feel guilty.

6. REACH OUT TO THEM

- Taking responsibility for keeping communication going is vital because contact with loved ones is very important. It will help you to maintain your relationship with them.

- Finding new ways to show you care can be really valuable for someone with CFS/ME as the condition can feel very isolating.

- Don't give up on them; if they are out of contact they may be having a bad time.

7. HELP THEM 'PACE' THEMSELVES

- Any help you can give your friend or family member to manage their limited energy levels, whether it is reminding them to take rest breaks or helping them to plan their days, will be useful.

- Keep remembering that they need to do things differently to avoid making their symptoms worse and have the best quality of life they can with the illness.

May, 31, friend of a moderately affected person, says:

> Encouragement is really important… Let the person know you are behind them and that you believe they can get better, even if it takes time. The recovery process can be

exhausting in itself, so regular encouragement and acknowledgement of your loved one's achievements so far is essential I think.

8. LET GO OF EXPECTATIONS

- Try to be aware of times when you are disappointed that your loved one is behaving differently, whether it is not taking their usual role in family events or not giving you as much support or time as before. These changes are likely to be because of the illness and they are probably not happy about them either.

- This is a time of great change for your loved one and you, and it can be an opportunity for new and positive developments in your relationship if you are prepared to be flexible.

Ian, 32, brother of a CFS/ME sufferer, advises:

Be prepared to make sacrifices in your expectations of your loved one.

9. OFFER WHAT YOU CAN

- Try to find ways to help if you want to, even if you are not sure what you can do. Just ask!

- Being honest about what you can and can't do for them is very helpful for you both and will help you to negotiate something that makes you both feel better.

- If you are someone who prefers to show your concern in practical ways, there are numerous things that need doing when someone is ill.

- If you can offer a listening ear then do so. Having people to talk to about what it is like to have CFS/ME can help a sufferer and it will also widen your understanding.

'Michael', 45, whose partner had moderate CFS/ME, advises:

> Being with someone who has CFS/ME can cause problems in a relationship. If you're used to a partner behaving in a certain way, doing a lot around the house, etc., you need to revise your expectations, and take as much of the load off them as possible. Above all you need to be patient, sympathetic, and put their needs first.

10. KEEP POSITIVE

- It can be very hard to cope with CFS/ME, for the person who has it as well as for their loved ones around them, especially as it is difficult to know what it will mean in the long term. Negative information and the losses that come with having the illness can make things seem hopeless. Focusing on what *can* be done gives everyone a sense of purpose and positive focus.

- Helping your loved one to keep positivity in their life through social contact, support and enjoyable activities will help them find a balance between the very real struggle and suffering CFS/ME brings and other aspects of life that they can still get something positive out of.

- Be patient both with the process of the illness or treatments someone may be following; with their necessarily reduced pace of life this is a very valuable support.

Jane, 33, severely affected CFS/ME patient, says:

> Take each day as it comes, no one can rush the recovery, and putting pressure on them is unhelpful as they'll be doing that to themselves anyway! Remain positive and encouraging with them. Focus on the positives instead of dwelling on all the losses and what the sufferer can't do; focus on the progress that's been made and the future. The past is history.

FINAL NOTE FROM THE AUTHOR

I hope there is something for everyone in this book and that some of the suggestions made help you support a loved one with CFS/ME. Whether you live near or far from your friend or family member, there are numerous things you can do. Just being there and showing you care is precious and can help us get through the hardest times. I wish you all the very best for the future and on behalf of your friend or relative with CFS/ME, I would like to thank you for all the help and support you give as they cope with this illness. As you have seen in the examples given, sometimes it is the smallest things that mean the most.

References

Action for ME (2006) 'ME – More Than You Know': Survey of 2000 People with CFS/ME. Bristol: Action for ME.

Action for ME (2007) Pacing for People with ME. (Booklet) Bristol: Action for ME.

Houdenhove, B.V., Bruyninckx, K. and Luyten, P. (2006) 'In search of a new balance. Can high "action-proneness" in patients with chronic fatigue syndrome be changed by multidisciplinary group treatment?' Journal of Psychosomatic Research 60, 623–625.

King's College London (2008) Information for Patients – Physiological Aspects of CFS. Available at www.kcl.ac.uk/projects/cfs/patients/physiology, accessed on 19 April 2010.

Leeds, A., Brand Miller, J., Foster-Powell, K. and Colagiuri, S. (2003) The New Glucose Revolution (Third edition). London: Hodder and Stoughton.

NICE (National Institute for Health and Clinical Excellence) (2007) Clinical Guideline 53: Chronic Fatigue Syndrome/Myalgic Encephalomyelitis (or Encephalopathy). Diagnosis and Management of CFS/ME in Adults and Children. London: NICE.

Nye, F.J. and Crawley, E. (2007) 'Chronic fatigue syndrome: altered physiology and genetic influences.' Royal College of Physicians of Edinburgh and Royal College of Physicians and Surgeons of Glasgow. Available at http://behindtheheadlines.com/articles/chronic-fatigue-syndrome-altered-physiology-and-genetic-influences, accessed April 2009.

Powell, P., Bentall, R.P., Nye, F.J. and Edwards, R.H.T. (2001) 'Randomised controlled trial of patient education to encourage graded exercise in chronic fatigue syndrome.' British Medical *Journal 322*, 387–391.

Ward, T., Hogan, K., Stuart, V. and Singleton, E. (2008) 'The experiences of counselling for persons with ME.' *Counselling and Psychotherapy Research 8*, 2, 73–79.

Williams, G., Waterhouse, J., Minors, D. and Edwards, R.H.T. (1996) 'Disruption of Circadian Rhythmicity in patients with Chronic Fatigue Syndrome.' *Clinical Physiology 16*, 327–333.

Resources

This section of the book aims to provide you with further sources of information for the subjects discussed in the book, and places you can go to for support or further understanding of CFS/ME and how it affects you.

BENEFITS/FINANCIAL SUPPORT

The following are specific benefits advice agencies. For impartial advice specific to CFS/ME see the 'CFS/ME charities' and 'Disability issues' sections for relevant organisations.

UK

Disability Alliance
Provides information for people with disabilities covering a range of issues including social security benefits and tax credits. They also run a dedicated telephone helpline for members with over 400 member organisations that are both local and national in their scope. They advise and lobby MPs on the effects of new and existing disability benefits.

Universal House
88–94 Wentworth Street
London E1 7SA
Telephone: 020 7247 8776
Email: office.da@dial.pipex.com
Website: www.disabilityalliance.org

The Department for Work and Pensions
Government department responsible for benefits and employment issues. See website or contact one of the specific helplines listed below.

Disability Benefits

For information about Disability Benefits including Incapacity Benefit, Employment and Support Allowance, Disability Living Allowance, Disabled Element of Tax Credit, and Disabled Facilities Grants and Community Care Grants.

> Telephone: 0800 88 2200 8.30am to 6.30pm Monday to Friday, 9am to 1pm Saturday.
> Northern Ireland: 0800 22 06 74

Carer's Benefits

Carer's Allowance is available to people aged 16+ who spend at least 35 hours per week looking after someone who receives one of these qualifying benefits: Disability Living Allowance (Care component, Middle or Higher rate), Attendance Allowance or Constant Attendance Allowance. (If working the carer's net pay must be less than £95.00 per week to qualify.)

> Telephone: 01253 856 123 9am to 5pm Monday to Thursday, 8am to 4.30pm Friday.
> Carers Allowance Unit: 01772 899729 (028 9090 6186 in Northern Ireland)
> Working Tax Credit Helpline: 0845 300 3900 (0845 603 2000 in Northern Ireland)
> Website: www.direct.gov.uk

Citizens Advice Bureaux
Free face-to-face and internet advice and support regarding benefits, employment, legal, disability, discrimination and financial problems across the UK – find your nearest branch on their website or by looking in your local telephone directory.

> Website: www.citizensadvice.org.uk

Ireland

The Citizens Information Board

Government website providing information on public services including benefits, employment and health issues.

Ground Floor
George's Quay House
43 Townsend Street
Dublin 2
Helpline: lo-call 1890 777 121, 9am to 9pm Monday to Friday.
Telephone: +353 1 605 9000
Website: www.citizensinformation.ie

US

GovBenefits

Government online resource for information on benefits and assistance programmes.

Website: www.govbenefits.gov

The United States Department of Labor

Information on unemployment insurance including departmental telephone and email contact details.

US Department of Labor
200 Constitution Ave., NW
Washington, DC 20210
Telephone: National Toll-Free Contact Center Monday
through Friday from 8am to 8pm Eastern Time by calling,
1-866-4-USA-DOL, TTY: 1-877-889-5627.
Website: www.dol.gov/dol/topic/unemployment-insurance

Australia

Centrelink

Government online resource including information on carers and sickness benefits, and an online application process.

Website: www.centrelink.gov.au

New Zealand

Work and Income
Government resource including information on carers and sickness benefits.

Telephone: 0800 559 009
Website: www.workandincome.govt.nz

Canada

Canada Benefits
Government website providing benefits information and benefits finder resource.

Helpline: Toll-free: 1 800 O-Canada (1-800-622-6232) or
TTY/TDD: 1-800-926-9105 available 8am to 8pm Eastern
time Monday to Friday.
Website: www.canadabenefits.gc.ca

CARER'S SUPPORT
UK

Carers UK
National charity offering support, advice and information to carers, including carer's assessments and advice on looking after yourself.

32–36 Loman Street
Southwark
London SE11 0EE
Telephone: 020 7922 8000 or to order publications telephone:
0845 241 0963.
Helpline (CarersLine): 0808 808 7777, 10am to 12pm and 2pm
to 4pm Wednesday and Thursday.
Email: info@carersuk.org
Website: www.carersuk.org

Carers Scotland
The Cottage
21 Pearce Street
Glasgow G51 3UT
Telephone: 0141 445 3070
Email: info@carerscotland.org
Website: www.carerscotland.org

Carers Wales
River House
Ynysbridge Court
Gwaelod-y-Garth
Cardiff CF15 9SS
Telephone: 029 2081 1370
Email: info@carerswales.org
Website: www.carerswales.org

Carers Northern Ireland
58 Howard Street
Belfast BT1 6PJ
Telephone: 028 9043 9843
Email: info@carersni.org
Website: www.carersni.org

Crossroads Care
A UK charity with local branches providing practical support for carers where it is most needed, usually in the home, using trained Carer Support Workers. To find your local branch go to the website or telephone.

Telephone: 0845 450 0350
Website: www.crossroads.org.uk
Scotland: www.crossroads-scotland.co.uk
Northern Ireland: www.crossroadscare.co.uk

The Princess Royal Trust for Carers
The largest provider of comprehensive carers support services in the UK. Through its network of 144 independently managed Carers' Centres, 85 young carers' services (see Young Persons' section) and interactive websites they provide information, advice, advocacy

and support services. In addition, the Trust also acts independently in the interests of carers through: research, consultation and policy development work.

Unit 14, Bourne Court
Southend Road, Woodford Green
Essex IG8 8HD
Telephone: 0844 800 4361
Email: info@carers.org
Website: www.carers.org

Ireland

The Carers Association Ireland

National voluntary organisation for and of family carers in the home.

Bolger House
Patrick Street
Tullamore
Co. Offaly
Telephone: 057 9322920 or 057 9322664
Email: info@carersireland.com
Website: www.carersireland.com

US

National Family Caregivers Association

NFCA educates, supports, empowers and speaks up for the more than 50 million Americans who care for loved ones with a chronic illness or disability to help transform family caregivers' lives by removing barriers to health and well-being.

10400 Connecticut Avenue, Suite 500
Kensington, MD 20895–3944
Toll Free: 1-800-896-3650
Telephone: 301-942-6430
Email: info@thefamilycaregiver.org
Website: www.nfcacares.org

National Alliance for Care Giving
An organisation dedicated to providing support to carers and the professionals who help them.

4720 Montgomery Lane, 5th Floor
Bethesda, MD 20814
Email: info@caregiving.org
Website: www.caregiving.org

USA.gov Website
Page of resources on government website offering links to information about care, support for carers, benefits and respite.

Website: www.usa.gov/Citizen/Topics/Health/caregivers.shtml

Family Caregiver Alliance
Provides information, online discussion groups, services, research and advocacy for carers including the Family Care Navigator resource for finding state by state help.

180 Montgomery Street
Suite 1100
San Francisco, CA94104
Telephone: (415) 4343388 or (800) 4458106
Email: info@caregiver.org
Website: www.caregiver.org

Well Spouse Association
An organisation providing support to wives, husbands and partners of the chronically ill and/or disabled including details of local American and Canadian support organisations.

Website: www.wellspouse.org

Australia

Carers Australia

Aims to improve the lives of carers by providing counselling, advice, advocacy, education and training. They also promote the recognition of carers to governments, businesses and the wider public. Independent carers' associations operate in each state and territory, see national website or call for local services.

> PO Box 73, Deakin West ACT 2600
> Unit 1, 16 Napier Close, Deakin 2600
> Telephone State and Territory Carers Associations: 1800 242 636 to find local groups
> Telephone Carer Advisory and Counselling Service: 1800 242 636
> Email: caa@carersaustralia.com.au
> Website: www.carersaustralia.com.au

New Zealand

Carers New Zealand

Providing help for New Zealand's family, whanau and aiga carers.

> PO Box 133
> Mangonui, Far North 0442
> New Zealand
> Telephone: 64 9 406 0412
> Email: info@carers.net.nz
> Website: www.carers.net.nz

Canada

Canadian Caregiver Coalition

Advocacy, research, local support information and resources for family caregivers.

> Email via link on website.
> Website: www.ccc-ccan.ca

CFS/ME CHARITIES
UK

Action for ME
Charity provides a range of services including fact sheets, telephone advice, local support groups, a quarterly magazine for members, and is active in campaigning for research and policy changes. Their website is a comprehensive resource for both sufferers and their loved ones.

Third Floor
Canningford House
38 Victoria Street
Bristol BS1 6BY
Telephone: Lo-call 0845 123 2380
Membership: 0117 9279551
Telephone support: 0845 123 2314
Welfare rights helpline: 01749 330136
Email: admin@afme.org.uk
Website: www.afme.org.uk

ME Association
The ME Association has nearly 10,000 members, and a large number of local support groups. It offers several services, including a quarterly journal, a 'listening ear' telephone service and advice on welfare benefits.

ME Association (England)
The ME Association
7 Apollo Office Court
Radclive Road
Gawcott
Bucks MK18 4DF
Telephone: 01375 642466
Helpline (ME Connect): 0844 576 5326
Email: meconnect@meassociation.org.uk
Website: www.meassociation.org.uk

ME Association (Northern Ireland)
Bryson House
28 Bedford Street
Belfast BT2 7FE
Telephone: 01232 439831
Email: jo@nimea.org
Website: www.nimea.org

The ME Association has regional branches across Scotland and Wales. Details can found on www.meassociation.org.uk, and click on 'find a local support group'.

25% ME Group
The 25% ME Group represent people who have severe CFS/ME and their website provides support, benefits advice, advocacy and campaigning on issues affecting people severely affected.

21 Church Street
Troon
Ayrshire KA10 6HT
Telephone: 01292 318611
Email via links on the 'contact us' page on their website.
Website: www.25megroup.org

Stockport ME Group
Group providing support for people with CFS/ME, and their friends and family, in and around Stockport, in the north of England. They kindly took part in the research for this book and provide a model service of wide-ranging support for their members including social events, meditation classes, regular meetings with invited speakers, topical information, a lending library and benefits advice.

Website: www.subn.org/stockport_me_group

UK Fibromyalgia

They offer news, benefits and legal advice, support groups, a magazine, and nutritional and exercise information.

7 Ashbourne Road
Bournemouth
Dorset BH5 2JS
Telephone: 01202 259155
Email: info@ukfibromyalgia.com
Website: www.ukfibromyalgia.com

Ireland

Irish ME Trust

They provide information and a counselling service as well as targeting individual problems on behalf of sufferers. They aim to create awareness in the general public and the medical profession as to the plight of sufferers in Ireland and contribute to quality biomedical research studies.

Carmichael House
North Brunswick Street
Dublin 7
Telephone: Lo-call 1890 200 912
International telephone: 00 353 1 401 3629
Email: info@imet.ie
Website: www.imet.ie

Irish ME/CFS Support Group

They hold regular meetings, often with guest speakers, in Dublin, organise a telephone network list, and produce a quarterly newsletter. They are involved in helping set up support groups around Ireland. They also raise money for research and increasing awareness of the condition.

PO Box 3075
Dublin 2
Telephone: (01) 2350965
Email: info@irishmecfs.org
Website: www.dublin.ie/irishmecfssupportgroup

US

CFIDS Association of America

Working to increase understanding, knowledge and support of chronic fatigue and immune dysfunction syndrome.

PO Box 220398
Charlotte, NC 28222-0398
Telephone: 704-365-2343
Email via 'contact us' page on website.
Website: www.cfids.org

Australia

CFS Support

CFS Support is a site for people to find local Australian support groups, advice and somewhere to have fun with other people in the same situation.

Email: cfssupport@aapt.net.au
Website: cfssupport.netfirms.com

The ME/Chronic Fatigue Syndrome Association of Australia Limited

ME/CFS Australia is an affiliation of state ME/CFS societies.

c/o ME/CFS Australia (Victoria)
23 Livingstone Close
Burwood VIC 3125
Telephone: (03) 9889 8477
Email: mecfs@mecfs.org.au
Website: www.mecfs.org.au

ME/CFS Society (SA) Inc

Provides up-to-date information on research into CFS/ME, campaigns for the rights of sufferers, provides information on quality of life and management strategies and supports community education into CFS/ME.

GPO Box 383
Adelaide
South Australia, 5001

Information and support line: (08) 8410 8930, 10am to 3pm
Mondays and Thursdays.
SA country callers telephone: (freecall)1800 136 626
Email: sacfs@sacfs.asn.au
Website: www.sacfs.asn.au

ME/CFS Australia (Victoria)
Information and support line: (03) 9888 8798
Email: mecfs@vicnet.net.au
Website: www.mecfs-vic.org.au

New Zealand
The Associated New Zealand Myalgic Encephalomyelitis Societies Inc (ANZMES)
National organisation providing information for sufferers of ME/ Chronic Fatigue Syndrome.

PO Box 36 307
Northcote
Auckland 1309
Telephone: (09) 269 6374
E-mail: info@anzmes.org.nz
Website: www.anzmes.org.nz

Canada
National ME/FM Action Network
512, 33 Banner Road
Nepean ON
Canada K2H 8V7
Telephone: 613-829-6667
Website: www.mefmaction.net

FM-CFS Canada
99 Fifth Avenue
Suite 412
Ottawa ON
Canada K1S 5P5
Website: fm-cfs.ca/cfs.html

DISABILITY ISSUES
UK

The Disability Rights Commission (DRC)
Have now transferred its responsibility for helping secure civil rights for disabled people to the new Equality and Human Rights Commission. The archived website of the DRC is still accessible via www.direct.gov.uk and has useful resources for information and support about employment rights from the Disability Discrimination Act (1995/2005).

Equality and Human Rights Commission
Providing advice and guidance to individuals and organisations on rights, raising awareness and informing legislation. Contact them by telephone for information.

Helplines:
England: 0845 604 6610
Scotland: 0845 604 5510
Wales: 0845 604 8810
Website: www.equalityhumanrights.com

Citizens Advice Bureaux
Provide impartial advice on benefits, legal and employment rights. Find your nearest branch by visiting www.citizensadvice.org.uk or by looking in your local telephone directory.

Ireland

The Irish Human Rights Commission
Leads on disability issues in Ireland, aiming to protect and promote human rights.

Fourth Floor, Jervis House
Jervis Street
Dublin 1
Telephone: +353 (0)1 858 9601
Email: info@ihrc.ie
Website: www.ihrc.ie

US

The Disability Rights Education and Defense Fund (DREDF)
Offering advocacy, education and information on disability law.

2212 Sixth Street
Berkeley, CA 94710
Telephone: 510-644-2555
Email: dredf@dredf.org
Website: www.dredf.org

Disability.gov
Internet resource providing information on employment, benefits, health, government programs, rights and housing issues.

Website: www.disability.gov

Australia

The Disability Information and Resource Centre
A free information service for the people of South Australia that is impartial, apolitical and non-sectarian. Aims to provide information that is current, accurate, relevant and timely, and in accessible formats.

195 Gilles Street
Adelaide SA 5000
Australia
Telephone: (08) 8236 0555
TTY: (08) 8223 7579
SA only: 1300 305 558
Email via link on website.
Website: www.dircsa.org.au

Disability Online
Victoria's Department of Human Services internet service for people with a disability, their families and carers covering a wide range of topics including health, benefits, work, social and advocacy including a service directory.

Telephone: 1800 783 783
Email via link on website.
Website: www.disability.vic.gov.au

New Zealand

Weka ('what everybody keeps asking' about disability information)

Disability information website, for people with disabilities, their families, whanau and caregivers, health professionals and disability information providers. Includes information on support, employment, equipment, benefits, travel and rights.

> Telephone: 0800 17 1981
> Email: weka@enable.co.nz
> Website: www.weka.net.nz

EMOTIONAL SUPPORT FOR YOU

Books

Kennerley, H. (1997) *Overcoming Anxiety: A Self-help Guide Using Cognitive Behavioural Techniques.* London: Robinson.

Gilbert, P. (2000) *Overcoming Depression: A Self-help Guide Using Cognitive Behavioural Techniques.* London: Robinson.

Silove, D. (1997) *Overcoming Panic: A Self-help Guide Using Cognitive Behavioural Techniques.* London: Robinson.

International

Local support groups for friends and family of people with CFS/ME are available in some places. To find out about services near to you it is best to contact your national CFS/ME or carers' charity or search the internet to see what services are available.

Befrienders Worldwide

Working worldwide with the Samaritans to provide emotional support, and reduce suicide. They listen to people who are in distress without judging or telling them what to do. See website for search facility for telephone helplines listed state by state in the US, Canada, Australia and New Zealand.

> Website: www.befrienders.org

MIND

Organisation promoting better mental health through online, telephone and local services. Website provides a useful comprehensive A–Z of common metal health issues including information on worry, depression, therapy, sleep, medication, stress, self-harm and suicide.

15–19 Broadway
Stratford
London E15 4BQ
Telephone: 020 8519 2122
MIND info line telephone: 0845 766 0163
Email: contact@mind.org.uk
Website: www.mind.org.uk

Living Life to the Full

A free online life skills course for people feeling distressed and their carers. Helps you understand why you feel as you do and make changes in your thinking, activities and relationships. Some of the things the course covers are: practical problem-solving skills; using Anxiety Control Training relaxation; overcoming reduced activity; helpful and unhelpful behaviours; using medication effectively; noticing unhelpful thoughts; changing unhelpful thoughts; healthy living – sleep, food, diet and exercise.

Website: www.livinglifetothefull.com

UK and Ireland

The Samaritans

Free and confidential telephone service offering 24 hour a day 365 day a year listening and support service for people in emotional distress.

Telephone: UK: 08457 90 90 90 ROI: 1850 60 90 90

British Association for Counselling and Psychotherapy (BACP)

They offer a 'Find a Therapist' facility to help you find qualified and experienced counsellors working in your area.

BACP House
15 St John's Business Park
Lutterworth
Leicestershire LE17 4HB
Client Information Helpdesk Telephone: 01455 883316
Website: www.bacp.co.uk

British Association for Behavioural and Cognitive Psychotherapies (BABCP)

They offer a 'Find a Therapist' facility to help you find qualified and experienced CBT therapists working in your area.

Victoria Buildings
9–13 Silver Street
Bury BL9 0EU
Telephone: 0161 797 4484
Website: www.babcp.com

National Counselling Institute of Ireland

Counselling training body also offering an online 'Find a Therapist' facility.

Walton House
Lonsdale Road
National Technology Park
Castletroy
Limerick
Telephone: 061 216288
Email: info@ncii.ie
Website: www.ncii.ie

US

American Counseling Association
Dedicated to the growth and development of the counselling profession. Website offers a 'Find a Therapist' facility.

5999 Stevenson Ave.
Alexandria, VA 22304
TDD: (703) 823-6862
Toll-Free Number: (800) 347-6647
Website: www.counseling.org

Australia

The Australian Counselling Association
National professional association of counsellors and psychotherapists. Website has a 'Find a Therapist' facility.

PO Box 88
Grange Qld 4051
Telephone: 0733564255/1300784333
Email: aca@theaca.net.au
Website: www.theaca.net.au

New Zealand

The New Zealand Counsellors Directory
An online resource of counsellors.

Web page: www.nzs.com/health/counsellors

Canada

Canadian Counselling and Psychotherapy Association
Represents the counselling profession in Canada and offers an online 'Find a Counsellor' facility.

16 Concourse Gate, Suite 600
Ottawa ON
K2E 7S8
Telephone: (613)237-1099 Toll free: 1-877-765-5565
Email via link on website.
Website: www.ccpa-accp.ca

FURTHER INFORMATION ABOUT CFS/ME
Books

Campling, F. and Sharpe, M. (2000) *Chronic Fatigue Syndrome (CFS/ME) The Facts.* Oxford: Oxford University Press.
A practical scientifically-based guide to the illness written by a sufferer and medical professional, covering causes, treatments, and self-help.

Burgess, M. with Chalder, T. (2005) *Overcoming Chronic Fatigue – A Self-help Guide using Cognitive Behavioural Techniques.* London: Constable.
An accessible guide to managing fatigue illnesses, including activity planning, pacing, sleep hygiene, managing the negative effects on mental health.

'Sleepydust'
A comprehensive UK-based resource maintained by people with CFS/ME that offers wide-ranging information on symptoms, management strategies and research, offering an email 'ezine' with regular updates on the latest news in the field and treatment reviews from sufferers. A video is available for friends and family that you can watch on the website to help you understand the illness.

Website: www.sleepydust.net

MEDICAL RESOURCES (GENERAL)
Patient UK
An internet resource often used by GPs during consultations that provides useful explanations of health problems – CFS/ME, anxiety, depression, etc.

Website: www.patient.co.uk

NHS Direct
Free NHS information service on a wide range of medical, service and treatment issues.

Telephone: 0845 46 47 (England) 08454 24 24 24 (NHS 24 Scotland)
Website: www.nhsdirect.nhs.uk, www.nhs24.com (Scotland)

MOBILITY

Disabled Living Foundation

A national UK charity providing free advice to people with disabilities, their family and carers about daily living equipment and mobility products.

380 Harrow Road
London W9 2HU
Telephone: 0207 289 6111
Helpline: 0845 130 9177, 10am to 4pm Monday to Friday.
Email: advice@dlf.org.uk
Website: www.dlf.org.uk

Ableize

Online directory of disability information, aids and mobility services. Find products and services, sports and holidays plus the largest collection of disabled clubs, groups and charities in the UK.

Website: www.ableize.com

The Blue Badge Parking Scheme, Shopmobility and Free Bus Passes for disabled people

These schemes allow people with disabilities that restrict their mobility to park in designated parking bays close to local amenities, have assistance when shopping and obtain free bus travel. Apply by contacting your local council, or see more details on eligibility on public services website.

Website: www.direct.gov.uk

NUTRITION AND ENERGY MANAGEMENT

Books

Leeds, A., Brand Miller, J., Foster-Powell, K. and Colagiuri, S. (2003) *The New Glucose Revolution* (Third edition) London: Hodder & Stoughton.
A comprehensive explanation of how to eat to maintain balanced blood sugar, an important skill when making the most of limited energy, including recipe ideas and a table of foods glycaemic values.

Ravage, B. (2005) *The G.I. Handbook*. Lewes: The Ivy Press Limited. Simple explanation and guide to eating with awareness of the effect on energy levels of different foods. Although written as a diet book, the guide can be used for reference for energy management.

PARENTING WITH CFS/ME

ME/CFS Parents
An internet forum/online community for mums, dads and mums- and dads-to-be who suffer from ME/CFS.

Website: www.mecfsparents.org.uk

Disability Pregnancy and Parenthood International (DPPi)
This charity offers support and advice on issues on being a disabled parent, via free telephone helpline, and also letter and email enquiries. Leaflets, factsheets and copies of articles on parenting with CFS/ME are available.

National Centre for Disabled Parents Unit F9
89–93 Fonthill Road
London N4 3JH
Telephone: 0800 018 4730
Admin: 020 7263 3088
UK Free Text phone: 0800 018 9949
E-mail: office@dppi.org.uk (office); info@dppi.org.uk (enquiries)
Website: www.dppi.org.uk

PREVENTING RELAPSE/STAYING WELL AFTER RECOVERY FROM CFS/ME

The Wellies Network
A UK-based support site run by people who are in recovery from CFS/ME ('Wellies') addressing financial, social, work and practical issues to staying well. It is a useful source of understanding for friends and family members who want to learn more about the ongoing effects of the illness.

Email: wellies-network@googlegroups.com
Website: www.wellies.me.uk

RELATIONSHIPS AND SEX

Relate

Provide face-to-face and email relationship counselling and sex therapy. See telephone directory or website for your local service.

Herbert Gray College
Little Church Street
Rugby CV21 3AP
Telephone: 0300 100 1234
Website: www.relate.org.uk

RELAXATION/SELF-CARE/ MINDFULNESS MEDITATION

Books

Kabat-Zinn, J. (1994) *Wherever You Go, There You Are: Mindfulness Meditation for Everyday Life*. London: Piatkus.

Mindtools.com

This website offers wide-ranging information related to the workplace but the section on stress management is a comprehensive free resource for ideas and techniques relevant to anyone living in stressful situations, including relaxation, meditation, understanding stress and cognitive techniques.

Website: www.mindtools.com, click on 'Manage stress' under the quick start menu.

Patient UK

Offers useful advice, information, online videos and resources for a range of relaxation techniques.

Website: www.patient.co.uk (under information leaflets menu, search for 'r' for 'relaxation exercises'; see also 'related resources' tab at top of page)

MARC (Mindful Awareness Research Centre)
Web resource from University of California, Los Angeles, US offering downloadable short mindful meditations.

Website: marc.ucla.edu/body.cfm?id=22

RESEARCH
UK

Support ME
An online resource of the latest research, articles and information about CFS/ME.

Email: info@supportme.co.uk
Website: www.supportme.co.uk

ME Research UK
A charity funding biomedical research into the causes, consequences and treatment of CFS/ME with a comprehensive online resource of research papers.

The Gateway
North Methven Street
Perth PH1 5PP
Telephone: 01738 451234
Email: meruk@pkavs.org.uk
Website: www.meresearch.org.uk

US

ME Society of America
Website offers references to sources of personal stories, research information, and information on symptoms and theories.

Website: www.cfids-cab.org/MESA

Australia

ME/CFS Australia (SA) Inc.
Website contains details of various research projects, diets, medications and therapies.

Website: http://sacfs.asn.au

Canada

National ME/FM Action Network
A non-profit organisation dedicated to advancing the recognition and understanding of ME/CFS and Fibromyalgia Syndrome (FMS) through education, advocacy, support and research. Website contains a library of the latest research.

Website: www.mefmaction.net

TREATMENTS, PACING AND OTHER MANAGEMENT STRATEGIES

The listed websites offer useful general information on managing CFS/ME. For information on local treatment options outside of the UK, contact your national CFS/ME charity.

Chronic Fatigue Research and Treatment Unit, King's College Hospital, London
A leading centre for the study and treatment of CFS/ME. Their website has useful resources about the history of theories about CFS/ME, Frequently Asked Questions, and downloadable information about self-help management strategies and treatments.

Mapother House, 1st Floor
De Crespigny Park
Denmark Hill
London SE5 8AZ
Telephone: 0203 228 5075
Website: www.kcl.ac.uk/cfs

Action for ME
Their website provides access to detailed online and paper resources about pacing and managing symptoms.

> Third Floor
> Canningford House
> 38 Victoria Street
> Bristol BS1 6BY
> Telephone: Lo-call 0845 123 2380
> Telephone support: 0845 123 2314
> Email: admin@afme.org.uk
> Website: www.afme.org.uk

NICE (National Institute for Health and Clinical Excellence)
Independent health organisation providing guidance on best treatment and practice for the NHS. The clinical guideline for treatment in the UK 'Chronic fatigue syndrome/Myalgic encephalomyelitis (or encephalopathy): diagnosis and management' was published in 2007 and can be read on their website.

> Midcity Place
> 71 High Holborn
> London WC1V 6NA
> Telephone: 020 7067 5800
> Website: www.nice.org.uk

'Sleepydust'
A wide range of online information on symptoms, management strategies, treatments and research, offering an email 'ezine' with regular updates on the latest news in the field and online treatment reviews by sufferers.

> Website: www.sleepydust.net

Patient Advice and Liaison Services (PALS), NHS, UK
Providing information about NHS services and treatments, support with concerns and problems. There are branches across England and Wales. To find your local branch, ask at your GP or hospital, or use the search facility on the website.

> Website: www.pals.nhs.uk

YOUNG PERSONS' CFS/ME SERVICES

Association of Young People with ME (AYME)

AYME (pronounced 'aim') is a UK-based independent charity dedicated to giving help, friendship, support and contact to children and young people with CFS/ME run with the young members themselves.

PO Box 605
Milton Keynes MK6 3EX
Telephone: 01908 373300
Email: info@ayme.org.uk
Website: www.ayme.org.uk

Young Carers Net

Part of The Princess Royal Trust for Carers offering online discussion boards, chat rooms, advice and local support groups for young carers.

The Princess Royal Trust for Carers
Unit 14, Bourne Court
Southend Road
Woodford Green
Essex IG8 8HD
Telephone: 0844 800 4361
Email: youngcarers@carers.org
Website: www.youngcarers.net

Index

acceptance of illness
200–1
Action for ME 19, 20,
22, 23, 42, 44,
137, 182
activity scheduling/
monitoring (pacing)
49, 137–9, 203–4
alcohol 133–4, 162–3
intolerance 162, 195
sleep problems 20,
107, 162
alternative treatments
143–5, 151
anger 91–2, 116–17
blame 14–15, 91–2
felt by family and
friends 58–9
anti-depressants 46
see also depression
anxiety 22, 113–14
felt by family and
friends 60–1
management of 40,
46, 102, 114,
117, 123, 124,
127, 150
appointments 147–9
aromatherapy 151

bedbound 27
bed rest 42

benefits and financial
support 168,
179–82
carers benefits 186
disability benefits 26,
168, 180–2
unemployment
benefits 179
body clock, disruption to
21, 43–4
body image 71–2
boom and bust cycle 25,
137
brain fog 22, 109–10
breathing, diaphragmatic
102–3
Bruyninckx, K. 45

cardiovascular system 43
carers
being the main carer
68–9
emotional support for
224–7
looking after yourself
93–5, 202–3
support at work 81
see also family and
friends of CFS/
ME sufferers
carers, helping the CFS/
ME sufferer with
caring responsibilities
185–7

cognitive symptoms
108–12
communication and
socialising
187–96
emotional effects
112–21
exacerbating factors
122–5
food and nutrition
156–63
housework, DIY and
gardening 176–8
individual recovery
strategies 136–
45, 149–52
making positive
changes 125–33
medical appointments
147–9
mobility and travel
168–76
money, employ-
ment and work
179–85
negative coping
strategies 133–5
personal hygiene
154–6
physical symptoms
98–108
preventing relapse
145–7
shopping 163–8

case studies
  CFS/ME sufferer as
    carer 186–7
  diagnosis 37
  doing things
    differently
    132–3
  early stages 39
  emotional effects 113
  food and energy
    management
    160–1
  levels of severity 24
  mobility aids 174,
    175
  pacing 137–8
  psychological
    therapies 141
  relationship changes
    73–4, 78–9
  shopping 166
causes of CFS/ME,
  possible 41–6
CFS/ME see chronic
  fatigue syndrome
  and myalgic
  encephalomyelitis
chemicals, adverse
  reactions to 194
children 76–7
  with CFS/ME 10
  parenting 75–6
chronic fatigue immune
  dysfunction
  syndrome (CFIDS)
  18
chronic fatigue syndrome
  and myalgic
  encephalomyelitis
  (CFS/ME)
  alternate names
    17–19
  descriptions of 28–31
  diagnosis of 36–41
  holistic approach
    14–15
  'invisibility' of 31–3

levels of severity
  12–13
possible causes 41–6
prevalence 19–20
stages of 23–8
symptoms 9, 20–3
chronic fatigue syndrome
  (CFS) 18
circadian rhythms 21,
  43–4
cleaning 176–7
cognitive behavioural
  therapy (CBT)
  47–8, 140–1
cognitive problems 22,
  108–12
colds 122, 194
colleagues with CFS/ME
  79–83
comfort eating 134–5
communication
  alternative methods of
    83–8
  in close relationships
    69–70
  importance of 197
  non-existent 88–9
  sensitivity in 89–90,
    194
  and socialising
    187–91, 195
  sufferer's reluctance
    to discuss illness
    33–6
concentration problems
  22, 111–12, 194
counselling 49, 94–5,
  140–1
Crawley, E. 45, 47
creativity 152

denial 35, 130–1
  on part of family and
    friends 54–5
depression 118–19
  see also anti-depres-
    sants
diagnosis 52–63

being the main carer
  40–1
difficulties with 36–7,
  120
overlapping conditions
  17–19
reactions of family
  and friends
  52–63
suspected illness 24–5
symptoms 37–9
diaphragmatic breathing
  102–3
digestive problems 44,
  157
disability
  assisted travel schemes
    173
  being disabled 26
  benefits 168, 180–2
  mobility aids 173–4
  visible 174
  at work 181, 182–3
Disability Discrimination
  Act (1995/2005)
  182–3
Disability Rights
  Advisors 181, 182
dismissiveness 54, 85
DIY 71, 176–8
dizziness 22, 104
domestic chores see
  housework
driving 168–70
drugs, illegal 135
  see also medication

eating
  appetite 21, 43–4,
    104, 157
  comfort 134–5
  for energy 160–3
  healthy 158, 162
  problems with 104–5,
    156–7
  social 159
  see also food and
    nutrition

emotions
    changes in emotional
        balance 72
    emotional outbursts
        91–2
    emotional reactions to
        diagnosis 52–65
    emotional support for
        carers 224–7
    helping with
        emotional effects
        112–21
    managing difficult
        63–4
employment see work
energy
    food and nutrition for
        160–3
    management 46–8
    see also pacing
environmental factors
    45–6
exercise
    for carers 95
    graded exercise
        therapy (GET)
        47, 139–40
    overdone 30
    and pacing 137
expectations 66, 204

family and friends of
    CFS/ME sufferers
    being the main carer
        68–9
    changes in relation-
        ship with sufferer
        64–7
    children 76–7
    common misunder-
        standings 90–3
    communication 83–90
    friends 77–9
    managing difficult
        emotions 63–4
    parents 75–6
    partners 69–74

reactions to diagnosis
    52–63
siblings 74–5
support for 93–5
work colleagues
    79–83
see also carers
fatigue 20, 28–9, 37–8,
    98–9
fear
    of being judged 35–6
    of life-threatening
        illness 38–9
    of relapse 146–7
    of ridicule 128–9
fibromyalgia 19, 219,
    233
fight or flight 22, 114
film and books 151
flu-like symptoms 23,
    29, 103–4
food and nutrition
    for energy 160–3,
        229–30
    home preparation 158
    problems with eating
        134–5, 156–7
    see also eating
friendship see family and
    friends of CFS/ME
    sufferers
frustration, feelings of
    59, 116–17

gardening 176–8
genetics 45
Glycaemic (GI) system
    160, 229–30
graded exercise therapy
    (GET) 47, 139–40
gradual onset 25
grief and loss 59,
    115–16
guilt, feelings of 53

headaches 22, 100

health problems, other
    82, 122–3
heat 123
helplessness, feelings of
    57–8
holistic approach 14–15,
    45–6, 136
hormonal changes 44
hospitalisation 27, 42–3
Houdenhove, B.V. 45
housebound 26–7
housework 71, 176–8
hydration 162–3
hygiene, personal 154–6

ignorance 56–7, 130
immune system 43
indifference 58
influenza 42
insurance 179–80
'invisibility' of CFS/ME
    31–3
irritability 91–2,
    116–17
irritable bowel syndrome
    (IBS) 44, 157
isolation 129, 187

jealousy, feelings of
    62–3
joint pain 22, 99–100

learning about CFS/ME
    201
Leeds, A. 160
lifestyle changes 70–1,
    124–5
    helping with positive
        change 125–33
listening 195–6, 200
loss, feelings of 59,
    115–16
love and protectiveness,
    feelings of 55–6
Luyten, P. 45
lymph nodes, painful 23

malaise 23, 103–4
management strategies
    for CFS/ME 46–9,
        233–4
    for difficult emotions
        63–4
    for energy 160–3,
        229–30
    for positive change
        125–33
massage 100, 151
medical
    appointments 147–9
    general resources 228
medication 46–7, 135
meditation 150, 231–2
memory problems 22,
    110–11, 194
menstruation 124
mental health 14, 44,
    118–9, 140
mild CFS/ME 12–13,
    68, 106–7, 188
mindful awareness 150,
    231–2
miracle cures 86–7
mobility and travel
    assisted travel schemes
        173
    buses 170–1
    driving 168–9
    long distances 172
    mobility aids 173–6
    parking 169–70
    resources 229
    taxis 171–2
    trains and planes 172
moderate CFS/ME 13,
    68, 107–8, 189,
    193–4
money 70, 179–82
    see also benefits and
        financial support
mood 44, 91, 127
    see also emotions
muscle problems 22, 47,
    99–102
music 151

myalgic
    encephalomyelitis
    (ME) 17–18

nausea 104–5
negative coping
    strategies 133–5
    combating negativity
        142
neurological system 43
NICE (National Institute
    for Health and
    Clinical Excellence)
    12, 37–8, 136
nightmares 22
nutrition see food and
    nutrition
Nye, F.J. 45, 47

onset of CFS/ME 25

pacing 49, 137–9,
    203–4
pain 22, 99–100
pain relief 47, 135
palpitations 22, 102–3
panic, feelings of
    114–15
parenting with CFS/ME
    71, 76–7
parents of CFS/ME
    sufferers 75–6
partner relationships 69–74
personality traits 45
positive thinking 141–3,
    205–6
post-exertional malaise
    38
post-viral fatigue
    syndrome (PVFS) 18
Powell, P. 47, 136
psychological health 44
psychological therapies
    49, 140–1
    see also cognitive
        behavioural
        therapy (CBT)

reaching out to sufferers
    203
recovery 27–8
    individual strategies
        for 136–45,
        149–52
reflexology 151
relapse 26
    prevention of 82–3,
        144, 145–7
relationships see carers;
    children; colleagues
    with CFS/
    ME; family and
    friends of CFS/
    ME sufferers;
    parenting with
    CFS/ME; partner
    relationships
relaxation
    resources 231–2
    techniques 102–3,
        150–1
relief, feelings of 61–2
resentment, feelings of
    62–3
role changes 70–1, 128,
    185

self-care 93–5, 202–3,
    231–2
self-harm 135
self help 136, 141–2
self-image 40–1
sensitivity to light and
    sound 23, 105–6,
    193–4
severe CFS/ME 13–14,
    68, 108, 189–91,
    193–4
sexual relationships
    71–2, 231
shame, feelings of 34
shock, feelings of 52
shopping 163–8
siblings 74–5
sick leave 81–2, 184–5
sick pay 179

sleep problems 20–2,
106–8
sleeping tablets 46
socialising 187–91
factors to consider
193–6
visiting 191–3
sore throat 23, 103–4
stabilisation 25–6,
145–7
state benefits see benefits
and financial
support
stigma 34
stress, persistent 42
sudden onset 25
suicidal thoughts 120–1
supplements, food 162
support
for carers 81, 212–16,
224–7
for family and friends
93–5
support, offering 204–5
swollen glands 103–4
sympathy, feelings of 53
symptoms 9
cognitive, support for
108–12
for diagnosis 37–9
emotional, support for
112–21
exacerbating factors,
support for
122–5
fluctuation of 25
overwhelming; sup-
port for 127–8
physical, support for
98–108
struggling against
131–2
see also individual
symptoms

talking, sufferer's
reluctance 33–6
telephone calls 188, 191

therapy 47–9, 94–5,
136, 139–143,
145, 151
tiredness 20, 28–9,
37–8, 98–9
toxins 45–6
trauma reactions 119–20
travel see mobility and
travel
treatment strategies
for CFS/ME 46–9,
233–4
for positive change
125–33
triggers see causes

understanding, lack of see
ignorance

viral infections 42, 103,
194
visiting the CFS/ME
sufferer 191–6

Ward, T. 49, 140
weight 134–5, 157
see also eating; food
and nutrition
whole person approach
see holistic approach
Williams, G. 44
work 70, 182–5
colleagues with CFS/
ME 79–83
support on return to
81–3
worry 60–1